Supporting Birth & Bereavement as a Doula

www.stillbirthday.com

Copyright © 2014 Christian Childbirth Services LLC

All rights reserved.

ISBN: 1500942162
ISBN-13: 978-1500942168

DEDICATION

To all those who brave to step with humility and love into the spaces where birth & bereavement meet.
May you doula your own heart.

CONTENTS

	Acknowledgments	i
01	Stepping Up, Stepping In	03
02	History of Doula	05
03	A Doula for Any Income & Any Outcome	21
04	What do I Actually Do?	41
05	Before the Birth: Medical Explanations	46
06	Birth Methods & Levels of Augmentation	81
07	Birth Plans	94
08	The Welcoming: Bathing, Photographing, Lactation Decisions, Postpartum Wellness	126
09	Loved Ones: Family, Friends, Providers	141
10	Farewell Celebrations	155
11	The Longterm Healing Journey	160
12	Bonus Pages	163

ACKNOWLEDGMENTS

The need to become equipped emotionally, psychologically and practically to enter into the spaces where birth and bereavement meet would not be necessary if mothers and families would not invite us to enter into such sacred moments. May we take a moment to acknowledge these courageous, vulnerable warriors of love.
More than anyone else, may we learn from them.

01.
STEPPING UP, STEPPING IN

www.stillbirthday.com

Dear Doula,

Maybe you're already a seasoned birth professional, or perhaps you are curious to see how it is to support a family experiencing pregnancy and infant loss. Your journey to this place matters. While we're here, let me share with you how I have come to this place.

I had been a birth doula for nearly ten years before I gave birth in the first trimester. And even with everything I knew about birth, I was entirely ill prepared to know what to do in such an experience. My interpretation of pregnancy has very much been woven with my spiritual beliefs, and as I looked upon the ultrasound monitor to see my lifeless baby bobbing in his waters to the movements of the ultrasound scan, I knew my baby was dead. Yet just as surely as I knew my baby wasn't alive, I was sure, absolutely sure, that God was going to speak life, breathe life back into my baby.

The ultrasound technician was talking but I was peering into the computer screen, in my mind saying "This is going to be THE coolest Facebook post, ever!"

The ultrasound screen was shut off. Darkness opened into a chasm, and I stumbled into it. I was going to have to walk this. I was going to have to make sense of this.

A doctor stepped in, grabbed me by my shoulders and said, "We need to get that debris out of there."

In time, my womb became home again to a baby. I sought the care of a midwife and had an extraordinary birth at our local birth center.

This book is not about the single experience of loss, because there is no such thing as a single experience of loss. This book shows how the culmination of our motherhood experiences shapes us, and even how our emotional, psychological and spiritual values shape how we define those motherhood experiences that shape us.

If you have ever been present at the birth of a living baby, I could bet my bottom dollar that your support has impacted a mother's bereavement journey. This book will offer guidance in supporting a family when first encountering death, when first encountering birth, and when supporting along the many stretches of the journey of bereavement.

02.
HISTORY OF DOULA

This chapter comes from The Invaluable Birth & Bereavement Doula
Source: www.stillbirthday.com/2011/08/01/the-invaluable-birth-bereavement-doula

-An excited mother meets with her prenatal provider to have her mid-pregnancy ultrasound and determine the gender of her baby. She leaves, totally devastated, as she learns her baby has a condition that isn't compatible with life outside of the womb.

-A mother experiences heavy bleeding accompanied by heavy cramping. She's only known she's been pregnant for a couple of weeks; she hasn't even seen her provider yet.

-A mother goes into unstoppable labor halfway through her pregnancy.

-A mother labors at 39 weeks, after a totally uneventful pregnancy, anticipating the birth of her live baby, when something tragic suddenly happens in the course of her labor.

What do each of these mothers have in common?

Many things. They are all mothers. They all anticipated giving birth to live children, and their dreams came to a shattering, abrupt, crushing halt.

And, through stillbirthday, they each can utilize a doula.

What is a doula?

Doula is a Greek word, which dates back to biblical usage. According to the New Testament usage, it meant someone who was willing to provide service to someone in need, so that the person in need would learn about Jesus' sacrifical love.

The Birth Doula/Labor Coach

Since its usage in scripture, doula has come to have something of a different meaning. Beginning in 1973 with the publication of "The Tender Gift" by Dana Raphael on the study of breastfeeding support in the Philippines, the term "doula" became associated with experienced women who come alongside new mothers while they are pregnant and during the actual childbirth process, to provide love, encouragement, information and support, in addition to continual breastfeeding support. These women are para professionals, and do not replace medical support (and are not to be confused with midwives), but come alongside the mother on her pregnancy, birth and early postpartum journey.

Aging/Seriously Ill/End of Life/Bereavement Support

In 1998, Dr. Sherwin Nuland, professor of surgery at Yale University School of Medicine and author of How We Die: Reflections on Life's Final Chapter, spoke at a conference hosted by the Shira Ruskay Foundation in New York of the Yiddish and Hebrew word for funeral, levaya, which means "to accompany."

One midwife (not to be confused with doula) speaks of her role through a Jewish "Taharah", which is a burial preparation that literally means "to purify":

"The act of helping a woman and her baby through their many transitions seemed analogous to helping the soul transition from this plane of existence to the next.

I performed my first Taharah, and it was more than I expected – more silence, more depth, more sensitivity. The concern of being with and touching a dead body left as soon as I entered the room. The midwife in me took over. The four members of our team worked quietly, with tenderness. And the energy, amazingly, felt the same as at a birth — a feeling of completion, a palpable sense of the soul transitioning and a humble appreciation of the privilege of being there." (source)

Inspired by Dr. Nuland, Phyllis Farley, chairman of the board of the Maternity Center Association in Manhattan, launched the Doula to Accompany and Comfort Program at the Jewish Board of Family and Children's Services in New York.

In 2001, this Board, with the support of the New York University Medical Center's Department of Social Services, began a doula program with this focus: rather than on providing comfort to mothers as they welcome in new life, this program provided comfort to those with serious illness, facing the end of life journey. (source)

Benefits of Bereavement Support

"Doulas provide stability in that they are a constant presence for the patient," said Rev. Marci Pounders, chaplain for the Supportive and Palliative Care Service and coordinator of Baylor Dallas' program. "Each [doula] is assigned to one patient at a time so that they may concentrate on that person's needs. They seek to relieve suffering and improve patients' and families' quality of life. Often just listening provides the ultimate form of stability." (source)

It is the goal of Rev. Pounders and the Baylor Office of Clinical Ethics and Palliative Care to expand their Doula to Accompany and Comfort Program to all Baylor Health Care System affiliates. (source)

Hogan's Grief Response Checklist and the qualitative data tracked positive outcomes for both the peer supporters and the clients participating in the Peer Support Program of the Canadian Mental Health Association Suicide Services in Calgary, Alberta. (source)

Comfort Zone Camp, through HelloGrief, notes the following benefits of peer grief support (groups) (source):

- Emotional and physical support in a safe and non-judgmental environment.
- Support and understanding from others who have experienced a similar loss.
- The opportunity to begin the healing process through sharing your own story and hearing the stories of others.
- Coping skills to help you through the most difficult days of your grief journey.
- Hope through companionship with people who "get it" and understand first-hand what you're going through.
- The opportunity to discover new traditions and ideas to keep loved ones present in your hearts and in your memories.
- Increased understanding of how children and other family members react to loss.
- Permission to grieve and permission to live a happy productive life.

The Journal of Obstetric, Gynecologic and Neonatal Nursing and Marianne H. Hutti, DNS, WHNP-C recognize the social needs of couples and families after perinatal loss, as well as the positive response in these families to social support, and encourage social support in addition to any medical care the bereaved family may need.

The Mayo Clinic notes that peer bereavement support can provide an emotional connection, relieve feelings of isolation, provide the bereaved with an opportunity to release powerful emotions they may otherwise keep to themselves, peer support can allow for the exchange of useful information ranging from disease research and new medications, to coping strategies even within the first year; additionally, it is noted that health care providers say that it can improve a participant's mood and decrease psychological distress. (source)

Results from Eric G Hulsey's Doctoral Dissertation, archived at the Institutional Repository at the University of Pittsburgh, of a study on childhood bereavement and peer support suggested that peer support programs can improve children's coping efficacy while helping to improve their caregivers' perception of social support. (source)

Dr. Phyllis R. Silverman, researcher and teacher. Dr. Silverman's research in understanding how the bereaved help each other led to her development of the peer-to-peer model for grief support.

Numerous additional research articles concluding the benefits of peer bereavement support are available.

Benefits of Birth Doula Support

Doulas supplement (not replace) medical support to provide the following:

- reduces overall Cesarean birth rate 50%
- reduces the length of labor 25%
- reduces Pitocin use 40%
- reduces the need for forceps delivery 40%
- reduces requests for epidural pain relief 60% (source)

These statistics were derived from live births outcomes. There are no current statistics on doula support for known fetal demise, but it can be concluded that doula support for such birth outcomes would reflect these statistics, although the degree of reflection is unclear. It is most certain that doula support for known fetal demise outcomes would not contradict these reported outcomes, including no harmful effects of such support.

One medical review of obstetric and postpartum benefits of doulas concludes:

"A thorough reorganization of current birth practices is in order to ensure that every woman has access to continuous emotional and physical support [doulas] during labor." (source)

Stillbirthday recognizes this to include mothers enduring pregnancy loss, giving birth to miscarried or stillborn babies.

The Cochrane Review of doulas and their benefits, along with a helpful explanation of their study, is available.

The American Academy of Pediatrics published a review pointing to continuous labor support not only lowering unnecessary interventions during labor, but increasing parental bonding with the infant – with the distinction between parental bonding and infant attachment, suggesting the newborn need not attach for the parent to bond. This would apply then, to babies born still, with no demonstrable attachment. This bonding can help facilitate healthy grieving. (source)

"Those of us trying to understand and be helpful to the bereaved are much more comfortable now with the idea that we always carry many relationships within us. A person does not always have to be present for us to feel connected. When the absence is the result of a death it is necessary to change the nature of the relationship rather than letting it go." -Dr. Phyllis R. Silverman (source)

Stillbirthday Birth & Bereavement Doulas : Trained Companions

Combining the benefits of bereavement support with the benefits of birth support, stillbirthday seeks to provide every mother and family experiencing pregnancy loss with compassionate and comprehensive emotional as well as practical support:

-SBD doulas can fill in the space between learning of a difficult diagnosis and the birth of the baby, supplementing perinatal hospice and medical support.

-SBD doulas can provide labor support prior to and during a miscarriage.

-SBD doulas can attend births at any gestational age.

-SBD doulas can provide postpartum support for mothers who've experienced pregnancy or infant loss.

-SBD doulas can provide services and support for subsequent pregnancies and births.

If you'd like to increase your knowledge of birth & bereavement doula support and earn the SBD credential, register to join our comprehensive training, which includes:

- prenatal education, planning and support for parents
- physical aspects of childbirth (stages of labor, process of birth)
- differences and similarities in aspects of childbirth by trimester
- navigating birthing options
- techniques for providing comfort during labor
- techniques for naturally aiding in progress of labor
- emotional aspects of childbirth which doesn't result in live birth
- guidance for home, provider office, hospital, and NICU settings
- physical postpartum care / recovery for the mother after birth
- emotional support for parents immediately after birth
- navigating the overwhelming time from the birth to the farewell (including things like hospital paperwork, medical examinations, funeral preparations)
- providing support for subsequent / "rainbow" pregnancies
- establishing yourself as a professional in your community / using stillbirthday resources and other resources

Gestation and Birth of the SBD Doula Program

In the week before official publication, stillbirthday has already enlisted the support of 200 doulas from every US state and around the world – and we are continuing to grow!

With the collaboration of perinatologists, social workers, nurses, midwives and doulas, we pieced together the first ever fully online, comprehensive birth & bereavement doula training certification program in the fall of 2011.

The Professional SBD

Stillbirthday Birth & Bereavement Doulas (SBD) provide support prior to, during and after birth in any trimester. SBD doulas are qualified to provide support in situations of fatal diagnosis, carrying to term, and NICU care. SBD doulas are equally prepared to provide comprehensive support in live birth outcomes, including subsequent "rainbow" pregnancies, and can serve as a labor support in all birth situations.

Click to view, print and distribute our hospital brochure.

Your SBD doula submitted a letter of intent to provide birth and bereavement support, has studied through a rigorous 8 week training, has passed with an 80% or higher on each weekly exam, has read and reviewed books relating to pregnancy, birth and child loss, has completed an investigative assignment in her community, and is knowledgeable in these subjects and more:

- the physiological process of childbirth
- how childbirth is different and similar in trimesters
- the importance of birth order and how it is impacted by loss
- how to support a mother in labor in any trimester and in any outcome
- how to help a mother build a birth plan, particularly in an expected live birth outcome or carrying to term
- how to provide immediate support when establishing a relationship prior to the birth isn't possible (such as unexpected pregnancy loss)
- how to preserve the fleeting moments the family has with their miscarried or stillborn baby
- how to incorporate personal wishes, extended family and siblings in the birth experience

The SBD doula is the standard of excellence.

Birth professionals who are not trained well in supporting families enduring loss may feel frightened, overwhelmed and generally ill-prepared to understand how to respond to the differences even as well as the similarities of birth in each trimester, or the labor when the baby is alive or not. Referred or transferred to a new provider or location isn't entirely uncommon, and can instill a message to the mother that everything is different because her baby is not alive – which is so very often an avoidable impression to make. There are many parallels of labor and birth and it is dignifying to keep these intact for the family however appropriate. Additionally, professionals in bereavement support can create an imposing feeling upon the family, as though their very presence looms the message of loss and death. It can be extremely difficult to try to speak through this. The SBD doula is equipped to serve in *all birth experiences*. Similar to live birth outcomes, an SBD doula can serve through the duration of labor, can identify sources of dystocia and can offer support in navigating the labor journey. At birth, the SBD doula can help facilitate bonding, which is different from attachment. Answering questions to what is "normal", how much "permission" each family member has in exploring their curiosities and feelings, and validating to the family are huge responsibilities immediately after birth that the SBD doula excels at. This we call the season of the Welcoming. And, the SBD doula begins to sense and can help facilitate the transition into the season of the Farewell. Having created keepsakes, creative and/or traditional momentos, assistance with photos and/or a photographer, the doula can speak in an appropriate way to the family about the extremely difficult stretch of the journey which includes their giving a professional provider the permission to have the physical form of their baby for burial or cremation. The average time an SBD doula might spend with a family at birth is approximately 8 hours. The SBD doula can also offer postpartum support in at least one to several postpartum visits, including attending the formal farewell if the family desires. Because the SBD doula supports all birth, providing doula support for subsequent, live-birth pregnancies can also be an extremely validating, healing, meaningful and joyful experience for the family.

You are invited to view the complete guidelines and curriculum of our SBD doulas, and to rate your doula who served you.

For a complete listing of all doulas, including those who are trained outside of stillbirthday but who choose to list with stillbirthday and comply with our Principles of Service, please visit our complete birth support professionals listing, or visit our listing of professionally trained SBD Doulas here.

If you'd like to become an SBD doula, visit our registration.

SBD Doulas who join through a networking partnership maintain the very high standard of excellence as an SBD Doula, as well as comply with the quality expectations of the partnering organization, such as Sufficient Grace Ministries.

SBD Chaplains

Requirements:

- Successful completion of the SBD doula program

- Letter of intent for our records

- Successful completion of any *emergency services* chaplaincy or *healthcare* chaplaincy training program is highly recommended but not required

- Ecclesiastical letter of recommendation on formal letterhead *or*

- Professional letter of recommendation on formal letterhead

- An extension of your doula community project, to include: a closer look at your regional groups of diversity (culture, religion, etc. and how you can serve these demographics through thanatological midwifery and chaplaincy), and, explain your local laws and the legal steps required, if any, following miscarriage, stillbirth and neonatal death as they pertain to transportation and repatriation information, funeral planning and specifically to home or "green" funeral planning. This should be a minimum 3 page report. Our *enrollment package helps with this*.

- Book review of The Invisible Pregnancy specifically as it applies to eco-thanatology.

- Book review of Ghost Belly specifically as it applies to the current challenges and support of birthing location options and outcomes.

- Attending a Professionals or Community workshop is recommended

- Signed agreement of the SBD principles of service both for doulas *and* for chaplains

The SBD chaplain provides options.

While the SBD doula supports as a companion through the birth and into the Welcoming and toward the Farewell, the SBD chaplain might enter into the space from there. Navigating laws and policies to best fit the families needs regarding an extension to the Welcoming, leaving the hospital or other birth space with baby, information regarding leaving the state with the physical form of baby, where to bury or cremate, the SBD chaplain provides options for the Farewell and can commit to seeing how these options might come to fruition for the family. The SBD chaplain can speak at the Farewell – funeral, or other ceremony that the family chooses. In these ways there may be a simple transition between serving roles as your SBD doula and SBD chaplain, or your SBD team member might serve in only one of these roles.

Unexpected Home Still Birth

Although the demographic is not notably large, families who plan full term homebirth but who endure unexpected demise face risks in bereavement that the SBD chaplain is sensitive to and capable of navigating. SBD chaplains are familiar with the dynamics of unexpected demise during planned full term homebirth and can help navigate the intensity by keeping the dignity of both the family and midwife intact when otherwise shame, guilt or blame might begin to proliferate and fester. The SBD chaplain seeks to honor the fullness of the reality of the life and personhood of your baby so that these factors don't become distractions to the healthiest bereavement journey. It has been proven that families who have blame or shame embedded into these earliest moments or scripted into these earliest memories are at higher risk of both complicated and disenfranchised grief in the years to come, while families who have the support of an SBD chaplain in these earliest moments, who have permission to honor their authentic feelings without fear of abandonment or blame, are much more likely to move into as productive and enriching a bereavement journey as possible.

M.O.T.H.E.R.

Midwife of Thanatology: Honor, Empower, Respect

If you are a credentialed SBD doula, and would like to further your education and deepen your involvement in your community, you are invited to consider becoming an SBD Chaplain. Click here to compare the SBD Doula role to the SBD Chaplain role.

Stillbirthday doulas have an extensive knowledge and skill set to support families in the spaces where birth and bereavement meet. Where the doula would supplement resources by inviting a chaplain to support the family during the transition from the Welcoming to the Farewell, the SBD chaplain stands to serve in this capacity. Becoming an SBD doula and chaplain both, means less transitions between different people, substantially reducing the incident of delayed or repeated support services, and it means a more holistic and uninterrupted level of care for the family.

Becoming an SBD Chaplain means having a proficient study in *thanatological midwifery:* a holistic (physical, emotional, social, psychospiritual) approach to death. This term is coined by stillbirthday, and reflects the advanced level even beyond our highly trained Birth & Bereavement Doulas, as the SBD Chaplains aquire a specialization in the care of the family and of the baby in specific regard to the farewell celebration of the family's choosing. Here is our list of SBD Chaplains or related content.

An SBD Chaplain knows how to mother the mourning.

Ways You'll Serve:

–Spiritual Support After Loss: As an SBD Chaplain, not only will you provide support in your community as an SBD doula, but you will serve your community emergency services departments, midwives and families (including those who you weren't already serving as an SBD doula yourself).

–Homebirth/Midwifery Situations: While there are hospital-based chaplains, your role is directly and immediately for the family and care team particularly in any out-of-hospital birth emergency, without delay. You will be contacted by your local emergency dispatchers, police, EMT or fire departments at received 911 calls in reference to emergency out of hospital birth, including neonatal and/or maternal demise. You'll be able to serve as a neutralizing presence in circumstances that include out-of-hospital provider negligence, abandonment or blame, by redirecting and establishing goals toward healing. (*see more below)

–Assisting with and Officiating Farewells: You will be able to serve your community through funeral planning, with a special emphasis on home funeral planning. You will be able to offer farewell service options to the family in accordance with state and local laws and the family's desires.

.

*In regard to homebirth loss, we at stillbirthday recognize three primary homebirth loss situations. In your role as SBD Chaplain, you may be called to any of these (explained below):

A.) Unexpected out-of-hospital birth, unexpected loss

B.) Planned homebirth, unexpected loss

C.) Planned out-of-hospital stillbirth

A.) In your community, this might include crisis situations such as a pregnant mother involved in a deadly traffic accident, domestic violence, or murder. It is important you have a clear understanding of what your role as an emergency services chaplain, an SBD Chaplain, entails.

B.) Because planned homebirth for expected live outcomes is on the rise, point B above is also on the rise, even if it remains a very small demographic. It is because it is a very small but rising demographic, that stillbirthday takes great care to note the potential for ambiguity and vast variability in how these losses are perceived and responded to, by families, loved ones, and care teams. This ambiguity can contribute to great conflict as the family searches for answers (particularly online) and is met instead by horrendous and even dangerous levels of cruelty, both by people in support of planned homebirth, and against it. These encounters can have a devastating and long lasting impact on families who are already deeply bereaved. Your role is in having an immediate and gentle presence, including offering a safe place for the family to unpack and diffuse their emotions without any bias on your part whatsoever, and to gather strong resources and support around them (including for their emotional, spiritual and physical needs), to walk with them as they begin to grieve in a healthy and healing way.

C.) Here at stillbirthday, we support exploring the possibility of planned out-of-hospital stillbirth as a valid option for families.

What You'll Learn

In your SBD Chaplain training, you will receive resources for, and will be guided in expanding upon, the following subjects, and more:

- Home or family directed funeral instructions

- Right of Sepulcher

- Statutes and codes for home funerals

- Preparing the baby honorably for visitation

- Instructions on filing, or getting support from others in filing, a Certificate of Death

- Transportation and Repatriation

- Green cemetary locations

- Funeral officiate

- Supporting your community as an emergency services chaplain with information from our Executive Team, Diversity Team and Prayer Team

My Notes

Stillbirthday Healing Timeline

2003

Heidi Faith:
- became pregnant for the first time.
- learned of pregnancy in Planned Parenthood.
- definition of motherhood largely interwoven with newfound faith.
- interest in birth doula work largely influenced by this spiritual underpinning of motherhood.

2011

April 19, 2011
- Learned via ultrasound 4th baby was not alive, wrestling with God, baby called debris.

June 2011
- Compulsion to help the next mother becoming almost unbearable. Cost for website was pressing factor. Web design plans on hold.

July 25, 2011
- "What, are you waiting for?"

August 1, 2011
- Officially launched the website stillbirthday on free platform

August 8, 2011
- At least one doula from each US state enlisted with stillbirthday and ready to start our training program. Doulas unanimously resounded with the core message of stillbirthday: a pregnancy loss is still a birth, and is still a birthday.

September 2011
- Perinatologists, social workers, midwives, nurses and doulas all gathered to contribute resources and information into the first ever SBD training program. It was $50.

2012

February 2012
- Online training began awarding 30 nursing contact hours.

Spring 2012
- Invited to other states and countries to spread our message of birth support for every trimester.
- Established trusting partnerships with similar focused organizations: SGM

June 2012
- First workshop for birth professionals in Virginia, hosted by Blessing God's Way.
- Paid platform for stillbirthday.

December 2012
- Published The Invisible Pregnancy

2013
- *Full schedule of workshops globally as well as online.*
- Began offering training in 4 sessions each year, rather than 2 sessions per year.
- Received exclusive permission from designer of Universal Breastfeeding Symbol to alter logo to represent bereaved mothers.
- Zero, M0M and DaD and Homebirth logos created.

Teams:
- Speakers Team
- Mentorship
- Love Cupboards

October 2013:
- Second annual October Remembrance event – First ever Hearts Release
Hot Air Balloon ride, releasing over 1,000 pedaled hearts with our babies' names written on them.
- Sealed official documents received from Reagan Library regarding Proclamation 5890

2014

May 4, 2014
- Opened The M0M Center

June 2014
- Credit listing written into Return to Zero, a Hollywood film

September 2014
- Credit listing written into Micro Birth

Teams:
- Chaplaincy
- State Representatives of SBD Doulas
- Diversity Team
- Seamstress Team / Legacy Swaddle

December 13, 2014
- Century ceremony / Love Wildly

(date) _____
- YOU received this handbook. You are part of the story.

_____ (your name)

03.
A DOULA FOR ANY INCOME OR OUTCOME

A Glimpse of the Journey

The following pages come directly to you from the Doula Handbook available at stillbirthday, and is a part of the welcoming materials of the training itself. It is included here just to show you how overwhelming it is, but also how important it is, to provide support to families enduring pregnancy loss. It is added at the beginning of the training as a quick reference for you in the future – and to see that the handbook barely touches what we will explore together (and it answers a question in exam 1 of the training!)

If you already own the Doula Handbook, you can skip through this section, although notes have been added within it to guide you as points of reference through the training.

You will see through the course of our training that we at stillbirthday not only want to prepare you to provide support for families enduring loss, but we also want to prepare you to provide support to families giving birth with expected live outcomes. The reasons for this are many, but include shaping you to provide the most comprehensive support in your community as possible. We interchange subjects in this training, shifting quickly from expected live birth outcomes to birth in any trimester. Some chapters have a stronger emphasis on loss (as does the inclusion of the Doula Handbook), while some, like chapter 2, have a stronger emphasis in full term live birth expected outcomes. Still other times, we navigate from loss by trimester in particular, to grief in general. Throughout the course of the training, you will find invitations for self reflection, which you are welcome but not required to share, and group discussion suggestions to help you create an ongoing dialogue with your fellow students. This classroom setup is not just a functional way for you to obtain the SBD credentials, but also opens the platform from which you can establish lifelong friendships with fellow students maturing into professional colleagues together.

From the Handbook

Safety/ Ways to Help: Before Birth

This section covers making the initial contact with the mother enduring loss, some basic tips on how to support her in the time between discovering the imminent death of her baby, to the time of the birth, as well as safety tips that should be kept in mind at all times. While knowing how to speak comfort to the mother in these earliest moments may not seem to be considered a safety issue, it truly is. Her emotional and spiritual safety may be in jeopardy and as the first point of contact, you have a responsibility to consider these needs and provide comprehensive support. Safety in all aspects as a birth & bereavement doula is a stillbirthday priority.

The Initial Contact

First, I will address your listing at the site. For certified live birth doulas who wish to list their services at stillbirthday, I am only listing names and emails, for several reasons. Stillbirthday.com serves as a way to shield the mother from unpleasant websites that may have at once been welcomed but now may seem hurtful to her. "Happy" websites, which focus on "happy" pregnancy experiences, seem to tuck a "sad" segment into them that doesn't offer the support she really needs. I believe it is important to shield pregnancy loss mothers from any websites which would be unintentionally hurtful to her. I am also not listing their phone numbers, because they've listed their services voluntarily, and listing their phone numbers can cause a number of problems that can simply be prevented by not having them published. This means that they need to check their emails regularly, and I know that can be problematic for some, but at the current time, I do believe this is the best route.

Getting the email gives them a moment to grasp the situation, decide the amount of involvement they can offer, and mentally prepare themselves for the work ahead.

As stillbirthday birth & bereavement doulas (SBD), your listing will be different. It will include your name, profile photo, a brief description of your personal and/or professional background (taken from your introductory essay), and any contact information you choose to display. I would encourage you to consider building a website for your services and letting an executive team member approve it; this will be addressed further in the final week of training.

When you receive the email (or first contact) from the mom, telling you that she is experiencing a pregnancy loss, you have time to assess the situation and prepare yourself. One thing you need to know upfront, and I will discuss in the section of attending the birth, is that pregnancy loss labor and birth, regardless of gestational age or how far along the mother is in pregnancy, can be very unpredictable. Early pregnancy loss, at home, can take anywhere from hours to days to even weeks to complete—including the birth of the baby, the entire placenta and all of the uterine lining. Do not tell the mother that you will commit to witnessing the birth, because you simply may miss it. I will discuss this in greater detail later.

Know that every pregnancy loss birth is different, just as every "happy" birth is different, and each one will be presented to you in different circumstances and events in your own life. Before you commit to a client, consider some of the following:

- What kind of support is the mother looking for? Did she specify how she'd like you to help her (most won't).

- Pregnancy loss births, regardless of when in the pregnancy they take place or the gestational age of the baby, generally take longer to complete than "happy" births. The timeframe for delivery can best be described as "unpredictable." An early miscarriage, for example, can be completed in hours, days, or even weeks. Active labor in miscarriage is marked by bleeding, but even this can come and go, start and stop, and, like I said, take hours, days, or even weeks to complete. It is not a good idea to promise to be present for the birth, because you simply may miss it. Mid-pregnancy (20-30 weeks or so) may allow for laboring and vaginal delivery rather than more medically assisted delivery (D&C or D&E). However, the labor can take hours to even more than one day. You'll need a very large timeframe to commit to the birth.

- What sort of support would be most beneficial to the mother? Would she benefit from a visit from you before the birth, phone support, you calling a support person (friend or family) and coaching them on how to support her, you attending a portion of her labor and possibly the birth, you attending a follow-up visit with the medical provider?

- What's going on in your own life at the moment? Would you, and can you, arrange for childcare?
Do you have transportation? Could arrangements be made that you can provide a certain kind of service for free, and inform the mother that if she'd like the support of your presence, that there would be, say, a small transportation fee? Be flexible, and provide what you actually can—and remember, keep it simple.

- Are you pregnant? Please, while you are pregnant, keep your support minimal. I request this for a number of important reasons: your "happy" belly can be a negative distraction from the love you are trying to offer, witnessing a pregnancy loss may generate sudden and overwhelming fear for your own baby, you may react negatively, and, the mother may be jealous. If you are pregnant, you shouldn't be afraid to approach pregnancy loss mothers. However, being physically present during any part of the process in the role of doula may be inappropriate.

My Notes

Because the suggestions and resources for supporting families where birth meets with bereavement are constantly changing, stillbirthday always publishes the most up-to-date resources and research right at our website. But in this printed version, you'll find spaces where you can enter in your own thoughts and notes.

_____
_____
_____
_____
_____
_____
_____
_____
_____
_____
_____
_____
_____
_____
_____
_____
_____
_____
_____
_____
_____
_____
_____
_____
_____
_____
_____

Suggestions for Supporting

From the list of support suggestions below, you can choose from any of the following—these are just ideas, and you can provide support in other ways if you feel they are helpful.

- Prior to even encountering a mother experiencing loss, consider how you might incorporate awareness about pregnancy loss into your birth curriculum or birth preparation materials. "My NICU" is one way that SBD doulas have to choose from as a way to begin to expose the idea of loss. Various cultural beliefs prohibit talking about death because it is seen as a kind of "jinxing," and others may simply be uncomfortable about in depth discussion. However, consider how local hospitals have NICU care to support in any outcome. Consider having a page on your website that is set aside to talk about your ability to support in any outcome. Include stillbirthday in your resources.

- Hire your local SBD doula on retainer. Designate a very small portion of every birth you serve, as little as $5 per client, for your SBD doula. This clears your mind to fully engage with every client, knowing that your SBD doula is only a phone call away from entering into any birth with you as your support for the family. This is especially valuable if you are not particularly comfortable in engaging very deeply into the areas of infant death and bereavement, or cannot invest into the full stillbirthday doula training. Your SBD doula serves as a back up to you, becoming an extension of your services to families. You can proudly say, "I can support you in any outcome. I have a team qualified to meet anything you may experience." By retaining your SBD doula through this very small financial agreement, he or she will already be compensated and can meet you in the births you need them. Your SBD doula then, agrees to be on-call for you, for virtually every birth you serve. Imagine, that level of commitment, for you!

- Phone support. Start by asking "What happened?" This allows, quite possibly for the first time, the mother to explain, in her own words, what happened. It allows her to process things, to voice them, to identify the reality of the situation. Let her talk it out; this is tremendously helpful and even healing. As she speaks, show active listening, interjecting occasionally with little comments so that she doesn't have to pause and wonder if you are even still there. Little things like: wow, oh man, that's terrible, that's so sad, and I'm so sorry, are appropriate. After she's finished her story, make sure you have a good idea of what has happened: how long the baby has not been alive, the kind of pregnancy loss she's having, how far along in her pregnancy she is, what medical recommendations or medical support she's had (you should never replace medical support, and even if a mother doesn't need medical support for her labor and delivery, and you are present, you need to act as a labor support, not a medical attendant, and should articulate your service upfront as compassion, not medical—the website explains this, but you should too), if she is currently in active labor (signs include bleeding, contractions, increased pain in lower back and pelvis).

- Get the number of a friend or family member. Coach them in ways they can offer support to the mother (and father). See the "Friends and Family" link at stillbirthday. If the mother needs transportation, please do not transport her yourself. Help her get a friend or family member instead. A friend or family member can also help arrange for childcare if the mother has other children.

- Arrange for a final ultrasound, if she doesn't already have one. This will depend on if the baby has been delivered or not, and how far along she is. Generally, babies show up best on ultrasounds if they have at least reached 7 weeks gestation, but even this is more accurate with a vaginal ultrasound, an option that may be limited, depending on her medical insurance. You can contact local crisis pregnancy centers, see if any have life-affirming ultrasounds, and if they'd be willing to provide your client with one. If the death of her baby was confirmed by ultrasound but she did not receive a photo, encourage her to contact her provider to ask for a photo.

- Refer the mother back to the website, particularly for learning about the different birth plans, and exploring her options with the birth plan that would best fit her needs.

- Bring over a small package of maxi pads (maxi pads are the one thing a mother never thought she'd need to buy for her pregnancy, she cannot use tampons, and even if she has some maxi pads, the first few periods following her pregnancy loss may be emotionally painful enough, without having to use the same maxi pads as during the birth of her baby), bring over a teddy bear (with a note that says "if you go to the hospital, bring me with you." If at any point her pregnancy loss needs medical attention, she should bring the teddy bear with her. Leaving the hospital (or office) with empty arms is heart wrenching. You could bring over anything else that would be just for the

mother, too, like a pretty journal, a candle, or anything else. You can keep your eye during the year for good sales of different items and store them until you need them.

- Offer customized pregnancy loss specific birth education. The website offers a great start, covering some of the basics like breathing, dilation and effacement, medical options, and natural options for birth, without including such things as bonding to the newborn that are often incorporated into other birth education curriculum. Mothers can reach this link from the same page as their birth plan.

- (for a full term hospital birth) if the mother has enough time to prepare before the birth, she can arrange to leave the hospital with her baby, and bring her baby to the funeral home. She will need to have already selected the funeral home and made arrangements both with them and with the hospital. You can call her hospital and funeral home yourself to ask about this before you present the idea to the mother so that you don't unintentionally disappoint her. Know that there are different state laws and different hospitals have different policies regarding this.

- Remind her she is still a mother.

- More information is available in our professionalism section, in chapter 8.

My Notes

Because the suggestions and resources for supporting families where birth meets with bereavement are constantly changing, stillbirthday always publishes the most up-to-date resources and research right at our website. But in this printed version, you'll find spaces where you can enter in your own thoughts and notes.

_____
_____
_____
_____
_____
_____
_____

Verbal Support

--Pregnancy loss mothers may be feeling a range of very big feelings. She may be feeling any of the following:

- total shock at carrying a dead baby
- both dread and longing for the delivery to be over
- deep shame/embarrassment/guilt
- jealousy or resentment at "happy" mothers
- failure
- love and pride at her child

For these reasons, it is important for us to be careful what we say.

- Encourage the mother that all of her feelings are right, even the ones that contradict each other.
- Don't mention your children if you don't have to, and don't bring them.
- Don't tell her she can "try again."
- For more tips of what to say or not say, visit the "Family/Friends" link at stillbirthday.
- Encourage her that "we're going to get through this—you're going to get through this."
- Don't refer to your "live" birth clients as "real" or "actual." Make a point to call them "happy" births if you must talk about them.
- If she's calling out questions from a broken heart, don't try to change the tempo with answers. "Why, why, why?" can be responded to with simple, "I know it hurts," or, "I'm sorry."
- It can be tempting to fill in any awkward silences with promises or answers. Don't make promises and don't give answers that you don't know or that wouldn't be supportive or encouraging. "This is the worst part of your grief" for example, is something that we simply don't know, and therefore shouldn't say.
- Give attention to the father too. A typically reported feeling of fathers is guilt and helplessness at not being able to take the pain away from the mother. Shake his hand, call him by name, and tell him that you are sorry.

Personal Safety in Their Home

Safety in doula work is imperative, and yet many of us take it for granted. Entering a client's home at any point in your relationship can be dangerous, and you need to use discernment.

Most doulas, for "happy" births, receive a phone call or an email, and then, without any further knowledge of the couple, they set off to enter their home. I do not. I have the initial exchange, scheduling our "interview," which takes place at a semi-private public location near the couple's home. Parks and libraries work great. I tell my husband when I am leaving, where I am going, and I call him as I am leaving. I bring pepper spray. Having the couple travel and meet outside of their home may seem like enough to hurt my business, when compared to the doulas who meet in the comfort of the couple's home. I am willing to lose a potential client for the (growing) possibility that I may have saved my own life. Doulas are taken advantage of all the time by internet predators, sending us emails trying to get our personal information. It really will not take long for these predators to realize that doulas can be too trusting. For this reason, I strongly emphasize safety and caution to all birth professionals.

When you call her, and you plan to meet her, again, I urge you to have extreme caution in entering their home. You will be entering into a situation filled with intense feelings and reactions, and either the mom or the dad may quickly become volatile or violent. When you are on the phone with her, ask her if she feels safe. You need to be aware that some miscarriages are caused by domestic violence. Some statistics indicate that women are 50% more likely to experience abuse while pregnant. If she says that she feels safe, and you feel that going to her home is a good decision, protect yourself with a few extra steps. Stop at the police station, with the address of the home. Ask if there have been any recent domestic violent calls from that location. Depending on a number of things, they may or may not be able to reveal that information to you. Explain who you are, and what you are doing. Leave a business card with the couple's address, and tell the police dispatcher that you will call when you leave the location. This may seem like a very dramatic step, but, every pregnancy loss is different, and even if there is the tiniest chance that this pregnancy loss may be a part of violence, I need you to protect yourself. Neither this website, nor the creator, can provide any kind of insurance to you. Your actions need to be made carefully.

Some statistics indicate that women are 50% more likely to experience abuse while pregnant.

Spiritual Beliefs

Death of our children can seem like a time in our lives when we are challenged by what we believe in life, death, life after death, and any intentional design or purpose to events in our lives. It is not uncommon for God (or a higher power) to be mentioned at some point during the pregnancy loss experience.

If you have a particular faith base, and the family doesn't, it can be extremely tempting to want to tell them all about your faith and/or try to evangelize them. Some of us are excitable about our faith, and we need to know that this is a very sensitive time and we need to exhibit self control. Your promises and witnessing can very easily be read as offensive, desperate, and extremely unwelcome.

If the family has a particular faith base, and you don't, it can put you in an extremely uncomfortable position if they ask you to pray with or in any other way engage with them. You can simply say that you are not comfortable with that, but that you'll wait until they finish.

If you do share a similar faith, and would like to pray for, with, or in any other way engage spiritually with the family, and the family would like you to, please consider the following tips for prayer:

- Get the father and mother together, and join hands in a small circle. Physical contact is important.
- It's OK to be nervous. You don't have to recite anything poetic or beautiful. Just speak from your heart. You should speak out loud and pray for both parents, even if the father wants to pray, too.
- Keep it simple. Pray for the couple's hearts as they endure this sad time, that they find healing and peace for their broken hearts. Pray that they stay connected and that, while their healing journeys are going to look different, that they can find their ways, individually and as a couple. Pray that they both find freedom from guilt.

More information regarding grieving your way will be addressed in chapter 7.

More information on how to support the family prior to the birth of their baby is outlined in chapter 8. More information about DIVERSITY is available at stillbirthday.

My Notes

Because the suggestions and resources for supporting families where birth meets with bereavement are constantly changing, stillbirthday always publishes the most up-to-date resources and research right at our website. But in this printed version, you'll find spaces where you can enter in your own thoughts and notes.

_____
_____
_____
_____
_____
_____

Ways to Help: During the Birth

At Home (less than 20 weeks gestation)

- Establish your boundaries upfront. You are not acting as a medical provider.

- At home pregnancy loss birth should only be for babies under 20 gestational weeks unless a midwife is present, because of viability laws. The midwife will be prepared with the legal information she will need. Please visit the section at stillbirthday for planning a home stillbirth for more information.

- Bring your doula gear—at least have it ready out in your car if any of it seems needed.

- If you bring a small gift like a teddy bear or even maxi pads, place it in a gift bag with pretty tissue paper. In the event that the mother accidentally flushes her baby (or chooses to flush her baby), she can cut a small square of the pretty tissue paper (about the size of a toilet paper square), write a note or a prayer on it, and flush it after her baby.

- Be prepared for a great deal of blood. Bring medical latex gloves and do not wear sandals.

- The mother should stay hydrated.

- Douching or enemas should never be used.

- Natural labor induction techniques can be used with supervision and caution. If bleeding increases to fill more than one maxi pad per hour, please discontinue immediately and seek medical support. Either ask that she have a driver take her to the hospital, or offer to call 911. Do not transport the mother.

- Sometimes in "happy" births, we find ourselves spending the night during an extended labor.
Please use caution and discernment when making decisions regarding the duration of your stay with the mother. Set limits that help the mother but give you a realistic timeframe and stick with them.

- Please familiarize yourself with the home birth plan at stillbirthday.com.

My Notes

Because the suggestions and resources for supporting families where birth meets with bereavement are constantly changing, stillbirthday always publishes the most up-to-date resources and research right at our website. But in this printed version, you'll find spaces where you can enter in your own thoughts and notes.

_____
_____
_____
_____
_____
_____
_____
_____

- Contractions and bleeding may intensify shortly before the birth. After the birth, the physical pain should diminish substantially. This would be a helpful indicator if the baby has been born yet.

- Prior to about 10 weeks, identifying the baby can be difficult. The baby will likely still be inside of his or her sac, which will greatly resemble the placenta pieces that are also being expelled. The placenta at about this time is the size of a pear, and it has very likely detached from the uterine wall from the pressure of the contractions. The placenta will likely not remain intact during the labor, and will be expelled in pieces that are about the size of large grapes. The home birth plan helps prepare the mother with suggested household items she can use to help retrieve any pieces during delivery, to examine and determine if they are her baby or not.

- Please do not retrieve any objects from the toilet. If possible, create a birth space in which the baby is held rather than slipping into the toilet bowl. We have resources in our early pregnancy home birth plan for this.

- Please encourage the mother to do all of the handling of the baby and placenta pieces. If you choose to help her search for her baby, do so without providing physical contact. The baby's physical form will likely be extremely weakened, and can be damaged easily. You wouldn't want to unintentionally damage the physical form of her baby.

- Be prepared that she may accidentally flush the baby, or that, if she is very early in her pregnancy, complete the miscarriage without ever knowing when the baby was born. Stillbirthday has a number of ideas at the "Farewell Celebration" tab that provide ways for the mother to validate the life and death of her baby without having the baby's actual body.

- Prepare yourself for what the baby may actually look like. Under the "See Our Babies" tab, there are photos of pregnancy loss babies from 4 weeks through 40 weeks.

- During her labor, she should not fill a maxi pad more quickly than one hour, at any point.

- Only immediately after the birth, this time is decreased, to filling one maxi pad no sooner than every half hour, for the first hour. If the mother bleeds more than that, there could be a piece of placenta retained in her uterus, and internal bleeding could create sudden, serious and dangerous consequences. Get her driver to take her to the hospital, or call 911.

- Will she bring the baby, and/or as much of the placenta as she can to the hospital? This helps with assessing what has been delivered and can help with any genetic testing. However, this is her choice, and generally she is not required to bring anything in with her if she chooses not to. The hospital staff will provide a detailed ultrasound instead to determine if she has delivered the baby and the entire placenta (and to assess blood loss). Know that the hospital may have policies that will dictate if the baby can be returned to the mother. She should ask about this before releasing her baby to them.

- E.R. times vary, but in most states, pregnancy loss patients get priority. The approximate time at the hospital may be about 3 hours. Decide if you will meet the mother and her driver at the hospital. If you do, you shouldn't return to their home with them afterward, but instead can excuse yourself at a point during the hospital visit.

- The "Farewell Celebrations" section at stillbirthday offers support at this point.

My Notes

At Office

- Make sure she has a driver.

- Do not drive the mother, but meet her at her home beforehand, or meet her at the office parking lot.

- Please view the office birth plan at stillbirthday so that you will be familiar with her options.

- Bring a teddy bear or other small gift for her to hold.

- Know that the hospital will, in all likelihood, keep the baby and placenta. They may be tested and examined. However, the mother can request that her baby be returned to her following the examination. Prior to the birth, she can call different local hospitals to compare their policies regarding returning the baby to the mother. If she wants her baby returned to her, remind her to request this at the time of delivery. If she will have her baby returned to her, the hospital will likely call her within 2-5 days after the birth. Her baby will be placed in a small container. You should warn her that when she receives this small container, it may be extremely upsetting to open it.

- The "Farewell Celebrations" at stillbirthday offers support at this point.

My Notes

Because the suggestions and resources for supporting families where birth meets with bereavement are constantly changing, stillbirthday always publishes the most up-to-date resources and research right at our website. But in this printed version, you'll find spaces where you can enter in your own thoughts and notes.

At Hospital

- Notify the medical staff immediately of the mother's wishes, in particular about the baby after the birth. What is that hospital's policy regarding releasing the baby for burial? Do other local hospitals share the same policy, or is there one more mother-friendly?

- Establish yourself as a labor attendant, just as in "happy" births.

- Bring your doula gear. Stillbirthday has a section entitle "birth education" that mothers can reach from their birth plan page, which has an article entitled "doulas," that has some excellent ideas (these are at the end of the article).

- The mother will likely need interventions. The "birth education" link expands on this. If you are a strong advocate of "every birth should be unmedicated," please know that this paradigm is not only unrealistic, but also unsafe for many stillbirth situations.

- Stillbirth labor is often unpredictable and often takes longer to complete than "happy" labors.

- In "happy" births, labor is triggered by a chain of events that include a message from the placenta to the baby to the mother. In stillbirth, labor is often triggered by the mother's drop of pregnancy sustaining hormones. Labor is commonly triggered within two weeks after the death of the baby (but not always).

- In "happy" births, babies actually help with labor, with their rotation and flexion. In stillbirths, the baby does not participate. This may be a cause of the general additional time of stillbirth labor.

- In "happy" births, the uterus is in constant contact with the baby, and the pressure from the contractions causes the fundus to press firmly against the baby. In stillbirth, this constant pressure is not always present. This may be a cause of the general additional time of stillbirth labor.

- Pitocin is often administered for stillbirth. Because stillbirth labor is not triggered by the "happy" cascade of hormones, and because stillbirth labor is not supported by the ways "happy" labors are, Pitocin is often the safest and most effective tool for stillbirth delivery. We should substitute with natural methods whenever possible, but work in conjunction with medical assistance whenever necessary.

- Particularly in very preterm births (20-30 week gestation), Pitocin is given in such high amounts that walking as a natural labor stimulant may be contraindicated, because of the risk of the placenta detaching from the uterine wall, causing internal bleeding to the mother.

- The emotional experiences of the mother may also be a cause of the general additional time of stillbirth labor. Her labor will be stressful, excruciating and agonizing for her. The mother's adrenaline, anguish and fear may override oxytocin, serotonin, and endorphins. Because her labor may be more intensive than "happy" labor, there is a high likelihood of using an epidural during labor.

- Provide all of the comfort techniques you know. Your support can supplement medical pain relief.

- Depending on how long her baby has not been alive, breaking her waters (AROMM) may be contraindicated because of the germ barrier and the potential risk of infection it may cause the mother. This is not always the case but is important to know.

- Occasionally the medical staff may need to use the EFM to check the contractions. It will pick up the mother's heartbeat, because the baby no longer has one. This may seem like a cruel joke to the mother. Be ready to hold her hand. It is not uncommon for the mother to also experience emotional dystocia.

- Because the integrity of the baby's physical body may have already weakened, episiotomy may be more likely, and forceps and vacuum extraction may be less likely. The actual delivery of the baby may seem to take a very long time. If this is the case, it is because the doctor is attempting to retrieve the entire baby intact. The weakened tissues of the baby's body can make this more challenging.

- In some situations, a Cesarean birth is deemed safest for the mother. If you have any questions about the doctor's decision, please ask to speak with him or her in the hallway. Bearing the scar of a stillbirth is a very emotionally painful situation for a mother, and if Cesarean is recommended, it is only because it is needed. Please do not attack the doctor, or pressure them to say something that could likely be very disturbing to the mother. It is highly probable that the doctor is shielding the mother from hearing any more tragic or offensive news, and you should do the same.

- Ask her if she wants to see her baby once he or she is born. Shortly after the birth will likely be the very best time.

- Depending on the initial appearance of the baby, the doctor may cut the cut the cord immediately, lower the baby or move quickly to another area in the room to clean the baby up. Ask the doctor ahead of time that if it becomes necessary for him or her to cut the cord, if they can cut it long, so that the dad can trim it later if he wishes.

Please view the different hospital birth plans at stillbirthday. There are plans for the following:

o 20-30 week labor o 31+ weeks labor o Cesarean
o twins with both stillborn
o twins with one surviving baby
o planned home stillbirth

- Prepare yourself for what the baby may look like. There are real photos of pregnancy loss babies at the "Gestational Age of Your Baby" link at stillbirthday.

- If you are emotionally able, ask the mother if you can hold the baby. Talk and sing to the baby, and tell the mother that her baby is beautiful.

- Do not suggest placenta encapsulation or consumption. I have contacted Placenta Benefits, and at this time, the risks of this suggestion far outweigh any potential benefits. The ability to consume the placenta depends largely on the condition it is in, and in pregnancy loss, it is quite unpredictable. Even if the placenta appears to be safe, the integrity and safety of its condition could be compromised. In addition, the suggestion of eating anything that has been in contact with her deceased baby might be tremendously off-putting and even considered strongly offensive or even vulgar to the mother.

- The mother will likely still experience the same postpartum hormonal changes including an increase in her oxytocin. She will likely experience love, awe, and pride at her baby, coupled with a mix of other feelings associated with her grief. Encourage her to work through all of her feelings, as each of them is normal and good.

• Help the mother navigate the immediate postpartum changes, including lochia (postpartum bleeding) and breastmilk. Ask if she'd like to pump and donate her breast milk, or if she'd like to dry quickly.

• If the couple does not have a pastor they know of that they'd like to be present, but would like to have a religious representative present to pray over their family, the hospital can contact a chaplain.

• The couple may want lots of family and friends and a pastor present after the birth. Help the mother look more refreshed by brushing her hair and getting her a fresh gown and linens. If your name was drawn for the giveaway in October 2011 you won a beautiful birthing gown from Bg&Co in New York.

• Most hospitals have a special refrigerator on the maternity unit to keep the baby in when the couple would like to rest, so the baby won't be taken to the hospital morgue until the couple is discharged from the hospital. Make sure of this.

• Most hospitals will make special rooming arrangements for stillbirth, allowing the mother to stay in the labor room for the duration of her hospital stay, or moving the mother as far away from other, crying babies as possible.

• In Cesarean stillbirths, most hospitals will make special arrangements, moving the mother immediately to a labor or a recovery room following the birth, and placing the baby in a bassinet next to the mother until she has regained physical control and can sit up and hold her baby herself.

My Notes

Because the suggestions and resources for supporting families where birth meets with bereavement are constantly changing, stillbirthday always publishes the most up-to-date resources and research right at our website. But in this printed version, you'll find spaces where you can enter in your own thoughts and notes.

_____
_____
_____
_____
_____
_____
_____
_____
_____
_____
_____
_____

Ways to Help: After the Birth

Choose from any of the following—these are just ideas, and you can provide support in other ways if you feel they are helpful.

- Phone support and resources given (refer to the "Long Term Support" tab at stillbirthday)

- Bring over a small gift, such as a teddy bear, a candle, a few frozen pizzas or other easy food so that she can continue to rest, an unofficial birth certificate for the mother to fill out (stillbirthday provides one under "Farewell Celebrations").

- You can encourage the mother to decide on the best time for the farewell celebration. If she's had a Cesarean birth, for example, she will need more time at home to recover. She can plan for any farewell celebration to take place after she is more physically well.

- You can encourage the mother that there are many ways for her to celebrate the very real life, and honor the very real death, of her baby, whether she actually has her baby's "remains" or not. "Farewell Celebrations" at stillbirthday has ideas.

- Encourage the parents that their healing journey has only just begun. The "Emotional/Spiritual Health" tab at stillbirthday offers articles on grief, and on explaining things to older siblings according to their age and understanding.

- Even for very early miscarriages, studies show that parental grief can be just the same as in any other age of child death (even adult children). The reality is, their child has died. They will need time to grieve. Pregnancy loss is rarely a single event, but is a long time journey to healing. Typically, the 4-6 month period following the pregnancy loss is generally reported to be the toughest emotional time for the parents. Talking and getting support helps.

- Refer the mother to the "Long Term Support" services at stillbirthday.

- Attend a follow-up visit with the care provider. Meet the mother at her home or at the office. Do not drive her. The timeframe can be a couple of hours, but the actual check-up (which may consist of an ultrasound and/or a vaginal exam and a consult with the provider) can be completed as quickly as several minutes. This follow-up visit is usually scheduled within a week, sometimes a bit longer, after the birth.

- If the mother has any questions for her provider, encourage her to write them down, to make sure they all get answered.

- Contact a friend or family member of the mother, to help coordinate the "after" support the couple will get. Refer the friend to the "Friends/Family" link at stillbirthday.

- Bring any photos you took of the birth, and have a backup plan if the parents aren't ready to receive them.

My Notes

When Your Help is Finished: How to Walk Away

Make it clear what the mother is permitted to do. If she called you for phone support prior to the birth, for example, and that is all the support you gave, tell her if she can call you again after the birth (and then use the "After the Birth" support tips listed earlier in this handbook). If you've finished helping her, and your services have ended, tell her that you are sorry for her experience (for her loss, that her baby died), and thank her for allowing you to offer what you could. Then, refer her to the "Long Term Support" link at stillbirthday, and tell her that you hope she can continue to find healing in her journey. Saying something very clear can be very helpful. Try "This is where my services end, but there are additional support services at 'Long Term Support' at stillbirthday."

04.
WHAT DO I ACTUALLY DO?

This chapter is derived from "How do I doula in bereavement?"
Source: www.stillbirthday.com/2014/02/05/doula-bereavement

1. Forget the Checklist.

Yep, the very first thing to remember, is that it's OK not to remember. Coming in with the checklist of "OK, I took pictures. I gave a teddy bear. Check, check, check, and now it's time for me to go." Even if you don't ever intend to give off this perception, it is one that many mothers can be keenly sensitive to. To help remember this:

2. Ask permission to open the window.

Whatever situation you enter as a doula, all you are given is a tiny window. That's it. Just a tiny window. There's always more to the story. There's always an unspoken need. Your job is not about being a success. It's about making a difference. Even if you believe you are familiar with a tradition, belief or decision the family has made, ask more about it. If the family says they are of a particular faith, for example, it doesn't mean that they want platitudes that are assumed to align with that particular faith.

3. Validation is always possible. Answers are optional.

You don't have to give answers. Not spiritual answers, not medical answers, not answers at all. But you can always validate. In fact, you should always validate.

4. Go Slow. Validate. Provide Options. Supplement Resources.

These are the 4 foundational points to everything. And to help you remember to keep these in mind, there's 4 simple words to start this off. "I want to know…." Ask this question in word and action, allowing the family to be the authors of their journey. Supplementing Resources is huge. It means that you don't have to know everything. Helping to strengthen the circle around the family – by incorporating people who can be an asset to the family, is substantial. Even with something as simple as "Tell me 3 people who love you" so that you can contact them on her behalf. Loved ones can utilize the support resources we've compiled especially for them – including how to honor during the Healing Journey. Utilizing stillbirthday as the resource for you is important, and offering it as a resource to the family is also important.

5. *There are 5 Seasons. And, there are 5 Senses.*

Seasons:

- Pregnancy (and everything up until the birth – this can include everything that went into the pregnancy)
- Birth (yes, this is a season all by itself)
- The Welcoming
- The Farewell
- The Healing Journey

The points above, about going slow, speaks to this. Don't shove one season into another. Birth, then Welcoming. The Farewell will come. The aspects specific to the Farewell will have time. Preparing with training as a doula, preparing with resources as a parent, is important. But emotionally, being present in the moment, in the season, is important. Right now, let's go slow. One contraction, one breath, one moment at a time.

Senses:

As a birth doula supporting during loss, it is especially important to be mindful of the senses during the Welcoming, because often if you have not established a relationship with the mom prior to birth, this will be the pivotal time to do this. With that said, it is substantially valuable to include the 5 senses during every season, as appropriate for the mom. You'll see that the earlier seasons impact the later ones.

"Check the Senses"

Whenever you're in a panic moment, of "Oh, no, I'm so scared, what do I DO right now?" Go slow. Take a look around, and check the senses.

- **Sight** – what does mom look like? What does the birth space look like? What can we do to create a peaceful, harmonizing, validating, special birth space? How can you capture the moments of this time, so that as mom enters into the next season, she can see the moments of love offered to her? How can you mirror back to the mother which season she is in? How can you reflect honor to the Birth and to the Welcoming? Can mom see you hold her baby? Can mom see you cry? How is dad being included? Can surviving siblings be included? Can parents spend time with their baby, really looking at her or him? In what ways might this be challenged? In what ways might you support this? You can use our birth plans for ideas, for birth in any trimester. What things will the family "see" as in, "perceive"? Will they see a birth certificate?

- **Sound** – what sounds are going on around the mom? Is she in a hospital? Emergency room? At home? What can you learn about the monitoring or other hospital equipment or policies? What music can you play? What words of affirmation can be spoken? Are there a lot of people in her birth space? How are they mirroring back to her the validation she deserves? How can you help ensure this happens? What terminology is being used to describe what is happening? How can using honoring words be validating?

- **Touch** – baby blankets, baby clothes, that are appropriate to the birth and welcoming experience, including size appropriate. All items specific to bereavement or the Farewell should wait, including, what will mom hold onto while leaving the hospital? Our postpartum resources give insight into this. What about how time and temperature impacts touching the baby? What are time barriers to spending time with, including touching the baby? How can you support in these things?

- **Taste** – what foods or tastes are pleasing to mom? Can she have a special meal before labor? Will there be a decision regarding breastmilk? You can use our postpartum resources for information on this. Can mom kiss baby? All of these things might fit into the taste category.

- **Smell** – giving a baby a bath who is not alive, can be anything from slightly different to substantially different from giving a baby a bath who is alive. Going slow is so important, and it is wise to rather invite the parents to do such special things themselves, although it can be entirely appropriate for you to do it too. Bathing isn't about taking off impurities from a baby, it's about the mom being able to look at her baby within waters, as a climax to bonding in-utero. It's about submerging the baby in waters of love, as the mother submerges in waters of healing. Using a special scent can be very meaningful. Likewise, spritzing the baby blanket or clothes also can be special. Oftentimes mothers will seal these items in Ziploc bags, to keep the scent even longer.

Now, what about issues of safety, or special circumstances, or financial or liability questions? I'd invite you to check out our full online training for the in-depth support into these and so many more aspects of birth & bereavement support.

I really want to reiterate about asking permission. You can show such great honor to the family by allowing them permission to author their own journey, at a time when so much can feel so enormously stripped away from them. Even if it seems a trivial thing, ask permission. This gives ownership. Empowerment. Authorship. Dignity. If you know that they are making a decision that you believe may complicate their journey later, such as not bonding whatsoever during the Welcoming, you can still go slow, validate, provide options and supplement resources.

"This is a scary time, and no matter what you decide, I'm here for you.
I feel compelled to tell you, that moms who have been here in this impossible time before you, who don't spend time in the Welcoming, as devastating as this time is, many have even more painful journeys later, past the Farewell, and if they could offer you any encouragement, it would be to spend a little more time in these moments. I'm here with you.
We're walking this together….."

My Notes

05. BEFORE BIRTH: MEDICAL EXPLANATIONS

The following pages are from the most frequently visited directly at www.stillbirthday.com. You can find all of the links referenced within these pages by visiting: www.stillbirthday.com/types-of-loss.

CHEMICAL PREGNANCY

If you have begun to miscarry, and hadn't yet been able to hear your baby's heartbeat with a doppler, your doctor might have said that you are having a chemical pregnancy. This means that it's a very early miscarriage.

Related: please read our Honoring Uncertainty

This very early miscarriage–or the name of it–doesn't make your baby any less real. At 5 weeks gestation, just about the time you may have found out that you were pregnant, your baby was about the size of a sesame seed. And, at 5 weeks gestation, your tiny baby's heart has already begun to beat. It's just too small to be heard on a Doppler.

While identifying your baby at this stage is probably just not going to happen, because of everything that is delivered during the miscarriage, including uterine lining and lots of blood, your baby is real. Your feelings about your baby are real.

You will likely have a natural miscarriage, or natural delivery. Rarely, artificial induction or a D&C may be recommended. You can learn about these different birth methods here:

- natural delivery
- artificial induction (medication)
- D&C

You are invited to share your story here as well: please remember that sharing your story at stillbirthday is a way to express your feelings and share your experiences with other mothers – it is not to diagnose, treat or answer any medical questions.

You might visit our farewell celebrations for ideas to celebrate your baby.

www.stillbirthday.com

HONORING UNCERTAINTY

Something happened. Something was… different.

You came to stillbirthday, you looked through our list of losses that we support, read a few of their descriptions – in particular, Chemical Pregnancy.

You looked at some of the photos we hold here at stillbirthday.

But… you're just not sure.

Everything seemed to happen so fast:

You felt pregnant, and then all of a sudden, you were met with blood.

Maybe lots of blood, and maybe with deeply painful cramping.

No real pregnancy test, there just wasn't time.

This was… something different.

There are many reasons why your cycle might change, even abruptly.

Sudden stress, including financial, social, or marital stress might impact your menstrual cycle.

Deep and longstanding stress might also impact your menstrual cycle.

Nutrition and self care also might have an impact.

Some mothers report a change in menstrual cycle after a big move, and there is something to be said for large sorority-type events that have a strong emphasis on women or motherhood. Examples might include women's rape survivor rallies, sexual trafficking fundraising or women's rights in childbirth conferences.

These things and more might have an otherwise unexplained change in your menstrual cycle.

Additionally, through our season of our menstruation, it is entirely possible, and even medically normal, to have an occasional menstrual cycle that is simply different.

And by different, any number of experiences might occur:

Your menstrual cycle might appear later, sooner, lighter or heavier than you usually experience.

If you have discussed these things with your doctor or midwife and still just feel unsure about what you experienced, please know that here at stillbirthday, we honor your uncertainty.

The feeling of uncertainty isn't easier and it surely isn't simpler than bereavement.

> Many mothers will resolve themselves to
> *"Well, I'll never know this side of eternity."*

And that can be a lonely, painful place to be. Please know, you aren't alone.

And in a time that seems so very fast moving, with answers for most things readily available, even for early pregnancy tests, it can seem frustrating and disappointing not to have a certain answer.

If you believe you may have experienced loss but don't have anything to "prove" it, we validate you.

You are invited to share your story here as well: please remember that sharing your story at stillbirthday is a way to express your feelings and share your experiences with other mothers – it is not to diagnose, treat or answer any medical questions.

You might visit our farewell celebrations for ideas to celebrate your "Maybe Baby".

BLIGHTED OVUM

A blighted ovum means that a fertilized egg has attached itself to your uterine wall, but the embryo (baby) did not develop. Cells developed to form the placenta and the amniotic sac, but not the embryo itself.

While a positive pregnancy test detects the placenta hormones (not an actual baby), finding out that you are pregnant can be the beginning of hopes, aspirations and joy.

With a blighted ovum, your body may display signs of pregnancy, and may actually sustain the life of the growing placenta for a short time. You may not know you have a blighted ovum until an ultrasound confirms it, or you may miscarry naturally before an ultrasound is performed.

The fact that a blighted ovum does not result in a baby can be equally–if not more–devastating than any other kind of miscarriage.

Finding out what to expect from your recommended birth method (listed below), and allowing yourself to experience healthy grief with a farewell celebration can be very useful and positive for you.

Please also utilize long term support services and emotional/spiritual health support services listed here in this website.

It is also very important to reach out, and tell others about your story. Please consider sharing your experience with us here and reading the stories shared here by other mothers who've experienced loss through blighted ovum.

We'd be so honored to learn from you and to cry with you.

Birth Methods:

- natural miscarriage

- D&C

We also hold photos of what you might expect to see or your blighted ovum to look like.

MOLAR PREGNANCY

There are two types of molar pregnancy:

Complete molar pregnancy. An egg with no genetic information is fertilized by a sperm. The sperm grows on its own, but it can only become a growth of placental tissue (hence a positive pregnancy test) and cannot become a fetus. In a complete mole, all of the fertilized egg's chromosomes (tiny thread-like structures in cells that carry genes) come from the father. Normally, half come from the father and half from the mother. In a complete mole, shortly after fertilization, the chromosomes from the mother's egg are lost or inactivated, and those from the father are duplicated. As this tissue grows, it looks a bit like a cluster of grapes. This cluster of tissue can very rapidly fill the uterus.

Partial molar pregnancy. An egg is fertilized by two sperm. If an abnormal embryo does begin to develop, it will quickly die because of the rapidly growing mass of abnormal tissue filling your uterus. In most cases of partial mole, the mother's 23 chromosomes remain, but there are two sets of chromosomes from the father (so the embryo has 69 chromosomes instead of the normal 46). This can happen when the chromosomes from the father are duplicated or if two sperm fertilize an egg.

Molar pregnancy poses a threat to the pregnant woman because it can occasionally result in a rare pregnancy-related form of cancer called choriocarcinoma (see end of document).

Molar pregnancy is assessed with a pelvic exam and ultrasound. The abnormal placenta mass will have a clustered, grape like appearance.

For these and other serious medical risks, the molar pregnancy is immediately ended with medical support. This is generally done with a D&C. Afterward, you will have regular blood tests to look for signs of trophoblastic disease. These blood tests will be done over the next 6 to 12 months. Your doctor will caution you that you will need to use birth control for the next 6 to 12 months so that you don't get pregnant. It is very important to see your doctor for all follow-up visits.

While a positive pregnancy test detects the placenta hormones (not an actual baby), finding out that you are pregnant can be the beginning of a hopes, aspirations and joy.

"The fact that a (complete) molar pregnancy does not result in a baby (or, twins) can be equally–if not more–devastating than any other kind of miscarriage.
Please be gentle on yourself and know that your loss is worthy to grieve."

- stillbirthday mother

Finding out what to expect from a D&C, and allowing yourself to experience healthy grief with a farewell celebration can be very useful and positive for you.

Please also utilize long term support services and emotional/spiritual health support services listed here in this website.It is also very important to reach out, and tell others about your story.

Please consider sharing your experience with us here, and reading the stories shared here by other mothers who've experienced molar pregnancy.

We'd be so honored to learn from you and to cry with you.

We hold photos of what a molar pregnancy may look like.

THREATENED MISCARRIAGE

If your doctor told you that you are having a threatened miscarriage, you should know:

Many mothers with threatened miscarriage go on to have a complete pregnancy.

It is better to find and treat health problems (particularly systemic ones) before you get pregnant than to wait until you're already pregnant.

Miscarriages are less likely if you receive early, comprehensive *prenatal care* and avoid environmental hazards such as x-rays, drugs and alcohol, high levels of caffeine, and infectious diseases. Being obese or having uncontrolled diabetes can increase your risk for miscarriage.

The use of *progesterone* is controversial. It might relax smooth muscles, including the muscles of the uterus. However, it also might increase the risk of an incomplete miscarriage or an abnormal pregnancy. Unless there is a luteal phase defect, progesterone should not be used.

The use of *false unicorn root* (or other herbs such as *cramp bark*) is also controversial. It is said to help "normalize" gynecological concerns with the uterus, including preventing miscarriage. This native US herb is said to help facilitate the release of hormones by the ovaries. Despite the claims to prevent miscarriage, there are warnings against using this herb in pregnancy. Please consult with your medical provider before attempting to use any herbs or other non-medical resources to sustain your pregnancy.

You may be told to *avoid or restrict some forms of activity*. Not having sexual intercourse is usually recommended until the warning signs have disappeared.

Remember A+B+C = abdominal pain, bleeding, cramping. These three *together* are signs of a probable miscarriage.

Are you experiencing [additional signs of miscarriage](#)?

We also have information in our [Getting Pregnant Again](#) section that may prove helpful to you in this pregnancy – things that are encouraging, and other non-medical things you might consider.

You are invited to [share your story here](#) as well: please remember that sharing your story at stillbirthday is a way to express your feelings and share your experiences with other mothers – it is not to diagnose, treat or answer any medical questions.

www.stillbirthday.com

INEVITABLE OR INCOMPLETE MISCARRIAGE

An inevitable miscarriage is different from a threatened miscarriage, in that with an inevitable miscarriage, your baby will most certainly be born via miscarriage.

There are two situations that result in an inevitable (or incomplete) miscarriage:

- Your cervical opening begins to dilate (open) and you are having vaginal bleeding (see our article on signs of miscarriage). This means that your body is beginning to deliver your baby.
- Your baby has not developed (stayed the same size) over a two week period. Your baby's heartrate may be slowing, or have completely stopped.

An inevitable miscarriage might be first discovered by ultrasound at a routine doctor appointment, or if you are experiencing possible symptoms of miscarriage you may visit your OB or your emergency room for confirmation. The emergency room experience is often considered very unpleasant, but it may be needed. If you visit your local emergency room, consider these tips:

- let the staff know immediately that you believe you may be miscarrying
- ask about their bereavement support, including staff and materials
- ask if there is a women's, laboring, or miscarriage room within the emergency room, or if you can be transferred to the labor and delivery level if that is what you'd prefer. Once on the L&D level, ask for a room away from other mothers.
- you may need to fill your bladder to help locate your baby on ultrasound. Ask about drinking water, and curling on your side, rather than recieving a catheter. If one is needed, ask about what to expect once it is removed (you may see some blood in your urine, and you may be sore for several hours or longer).
- if you give birth to your baby in the emergency room, inquire of your personal options. Visit our early pregnancy hospital birth plan for more details. Understand navigating hospital policies, including genetic testing, returning your baby's physical form back to you after any testing, and any other questions you have.

If your baby is *younger* than about 12 weeks gestation, you may be given three options for delivery:
- natural delivery
- artificial induction (medication)
- D&C

If your baby is *older* than about 12 weeks gestation (about the beginning of the second trimester), you may be given these options for delivery:

- artificial induction (medication)
- D&C
- D&E

You are invited to share your story here as well: please remember that sharing your story at stillbirthday is a way to express your feelings and share your experiences with other mothers – it is not to diagnose, treat or answer any medical questions.

You might visit our farewell celebrations for ideas to celebrate your baby.

MISSED OR SILENT MISCARRIAGE

If your doctor told you that your baby's heart has stopped beating, you may be experiencing a missed miscarriage or an incomplete miscarriage.

You may have just found out that your baby's heart actually stopped beating several days ago (or a couple of weeks ago) and you are just now beginning to see the earliest signs of delivery (see symptoms of a miscarriage for a complete listing, but includes seeing blood and/or pieces of tissue passing from your vagina).

A missed miscarriage occurs when your baby has already died, but the actual birthing process either has not yet begun or isn't fully complete.

If your baby is *younger* than about 12 weeks gestation, you may be given three options for delivery:
- natural delivery
- artificial induction (medication)
- D&C

If your baby is *older* than about 12 weeks gestation (about the beginning of the second trimester), you may be given these options for delivery:
- artificial induction (medication)
- D&C
- D&E

You are invited to share your story here as well: please remember that sharing your story at stillbirthday is a way to express your feelings and share your experiences with other mothers – it is not to diagnose, treat or answer any medical questions.

You might visit our farewell celebrations for ideas to celebrate your baby.

COMPLETE MISCARRIAGE

This means that the baby has already been delivered, and the *entire* uterine lining and placenta have also been expelled.

This means that you are no longer pregnant.

If your pregnancy was very early, you can learn more about what happened from the natural miscarriage article.

Please visit these pages for additional support:

- Taking care of your emotional/spiritual health.
- You can still honor your baby, even if your miscarriage was some time ago. Please visit our farewell celebrations article for ideas.
- Please consider sharing your story with us.
- We also have a listing of long term support services.

LIVE MISCARRIAGE

OR, BORN ALIVE PRIOR TO VIABILITY

When a baby dies in the first 28 days of life after birth, it is called "neonatal death".

Because by most calculations a baby is considered viable in or after the 24th week of pregnancy, technically a stillborn baby who is born live, even for an extremely short time past delivery, may also be considered under the "neonatal death" category.

There is no such category for the unique situation in which a baby born via miscarriage either is or appears to be alive for seconds or even minutes after the birth.

Because there is no such technical category, but because parents who experience this unique and extremely special situation wish to have their baby's experiences validated, stillbirthday has identified this situation as "live miscarriage".

A live miscarriage may be most likely to occur the closer the baby is to reaching viability status (perhaps 16 weeks and older).

In a live miscarriage, immediately after the delivery, the baby may curl his or her fingers around the parents' finger, may either appear to take a breath (as air is pushed into his or her body, particularly when moved), or he or she may indeed take an actual breath.

Witnessing such movements or signs of life can either be alarming to parents, or, for others, can be extremely validating and profoundly significant.

For this reason, stillbirthday wishes to validate this rare but important experience by naming it "live miscarriage".

You won't know if your baby will display moments of signs of life, until after your experience is over and your baby is born. Please do not allow this to change the course of your birth plans, if your birth plans are medically necessary. Here are stories shared by mothers who've experienced a live miscarriage.
The following information continues to give you support through the miscarriage process:

If your baby is *younger* than about 12 weeks gestation, you may be given three options for delivery:
- natural delivery
- artificial induction (medication)
- D&C

If your baby is *older* than about 12 weeks gestation (about the beginning of the second trimester), you may be given these options for delivery:

- artificial induction (medication)
- D&C
- D&E

You are invited to share your story here as well: please remember that sharing your story at stillbirthday is a way to express your feelings and share your experiences with other mothers – it is not to diagnose, treat or answer any medical questions.

You might visit our farewell celebrations for ideas to celebrate your baby.

VANISHING TWIN OR PAPYRACEUS

"Vanishing Twin Syndrome" may occurs when a mother miscarries one of the twins she is pregnant with. If the miscarriage happens *in the first trimester*, neither you nor your other baby should have any clinical signs or symptoms. The surviving twin usually still has an excellent probability of resulting in a full pregnancy and live birth, but it depends on the factors that contributed to the death of the other twin.

When a baby dies *after about eight weeks*, this baby and his or her placenta may likely be compressed from the pressure of the growth by the surviving twin; this is known as fetus papyraceus or papyrus. Generally, what is being compressed is the water that holds the small baby's soft structure while developing in the womb. Your doctor may inform you that your body has "reabsorbed" this water (or the baby), which might be *very* painful to hear. Because the baby's tiny tissues are no longer alive, your body may recognize your baby as a wound and begin to heal this wound by embracing the dead tissue to prevent it from further harming your body. You might consider something of like a scrape on your arm that your body scabs to heal. In this way, even your womb testifies to the painful experience you are going through.

It is possible that fetus papyraceus can occur in a singleton or a multiples pregnancy.

With twins, while both twins may be delivered, you should know what to expect to see if you want to be able to see the twin that has died (his or her physical form will likely be flattened and developmentally incomplete). If the twin died in the second or third trimester, there are increased risks to your other baby, including a possibility of having cerebral palsy and death. These risks depend on if the babies shared a placenta, or each had their own. For this reason, your doctor may suggest artificially inducing your labor prior to reaching full term.

You can view a photo of twins, shared by a courageous stillbirthday mother, one born alive and the other who died via fetus papyraceus, here.

Your doctor will discuss with you the possible need to induce delivery of your twins, and the likelihood of this baby's survival.

Please visit the specialized birth planning for giving birth to multiples (when one **or** both are still).

You are invited to share your story here as well: please remember that sharing your story at stillbirthday is a way to express your feelings and share your experiences with other mothers – it is not to diagnose, treat or answer any medical questions.

You might visit our farewell celebrations for ideas to celebrate your baby.

TWINS, MULTIPLES, HIGHER ORDER MULTIPLES

Also see our informational article on Vanishing Twin.

If you haven't done so already, please consider transferring your medical care to a Multiples Birth Specialist.

Please visit any of our specialized birth plans for giving birth to twins or multiples (when one or more are still) which also includes additional resources regarding multiples pregnancy. You might also visit our rainbow birth plan, as many mothers refer to their surviving multiple/s as rainbow babies.

Are you a mother who has endured a loss or losses involving a multiples pregnancy? Are you a surviving multiple? You are invited to share your story here.

You might visit our farewell celebrations for ideas to celebrate your baby or babies who are not alive.

www.stillbirthday.com

SELECTIVE REDUCTION OR TERMINATION FOR MEDICAL REASONS (TFMR)

Selective Reduction is a difficult decision families may face when pregnant with multiples. If one or more multiple potentially pose a danger to the health or wellbeing of the mother and/or siblings, the pressure to face this difficult decision may be even greater.

Because there are many different facets to such a difficult decision, we've divided them here to start with a general platform, simply to remind you that very fact – that there are many facets to such a difficult decision.

Regarding Loss after Medically Assisted Conception
- Loss after ART

Regarding Selective Reduction *specifically*

Here are external links to resources that are specific to selective reduction:
- In *Embracing Laura*, Martha Wegner-Hay tells her story of grief and joy after discovering she was pregnant with twins, that one twin would not survive, and giving birth to her healthy son, David. After being told that one of her twins had almost no chance of survival and that the sick baby could affect the chance of survival of the healthy twin, Wegner-Hay and her family made the difficult choice of selective reduction. *Embracing Laura* tells of the wrenching collision of sadness at Laura's death, and the joyous experience of David's healthy birth.
- Outside the Circle of Grief

Regarding Decisions & Loss
- In a deep desire to be sensitive, one of the facets of such a decision does include TFMR (termination for medical reasons), the intentional termination of life of one or more of the babies, and so with this introduction to this facet you might visit our starting place for elective abortion as it does hold information that may be applied into the very specific situation of TFMR such as selective reduction as well.

Regarding NICU
- The NICU can be a difficult place to be in, emotionally, for any reason you may be there. Our NICU support resources are here to help.

Regarding Multiples
- Here is our start page regarding multiples, which links to additional outside resources for pregnancy challenges and support, birth plans and bereavement support.

www.stillbirthday.com

ELECTIVE ABORTION

For every reason you may be here at this page, know this one thing:
you are loved.

A Glimpse of Grief:

While this website provides support to mothers who are already enduring the actualized or inevitable death of their baby via pregnancy & infant loss, this article begins by serving mothers facing elective abortion, in hopes that if there truly is *any* choice whatsoever, you won't *have* to need the sort of grief support the rest of this website provides, because grief is real, it can be hard, and it can be a part of your story for the rest of your life. There can be tremendous hope, healing and joy in grief, but these things may not ever entirely fill the chasm.

When a baby dies for any reason, mothers may grieve for them. It is an ongoing process of healing. The grief that mothers who have experienced elective abortion face can become compounded by a guilt that mothers who have *not* faced a decision about the duration of life in-utero may not share (knowledgeisempowering.com). This intense struggle impacts many aspects of the mother's life: the post abortive mother may be at an increased risk for depression and physical health risks associated directly and indirectly with the elective abortion decision (afterabortion.org)

Loss After Deciding to Continue – *Were you at one point in your pregnancy vulnerable to considering elective abortion, determined to continue the pregnancy, and then endured an unexpected pregnancy loss? This particular experience can create complex feelings of guilt, shame and confusion. Consider this: in any fleeting moment during the elective abortion and birth processes, a mother may face intense regret, and a change of heart and mind that feels like the experience is robbing her completely. Please, be gentle on yourself.*

You can also visit our types of pregnancy loss list to get support specific to the type of loss and birth method you are experiencing, and consider sharing your story here, so that other mothers enduring this experience after you will find validation in their complex feelings of experiencing unexpected loss after determining to continue a vulnerable pregnancy.

Possible Pre-Abortion Support:

Here is a list of the most common reasons mothers may face an elective abortion decision, along with a few resources that may be of benefit to the challenges presented. Following these alternative resource options, there are support resources listed for you for the journey after facing this enormously complex, deeply vulnerable decision.

When you are faced with making a decision regarding the duration of life in-utero, any decision you make (parenting through elective abortion, adoption, or rearing), having had to face the decision itself can be excruciating and even traumatic. Reaffirming that you are intrinsically worthy of respect, dignity and love is vital.

You are worthy. You are worthy.

Challenges & Support:

"I just don't think I can parent."

Possible Options:

Our [Birth & Bereavement Doulas](#) can offer birth education, birth support, and early parenting preparation, including supplementing additional resources.

There are several different kinds of parenting resources available in every community, including free classes at hospitals, and library books on the topic.

[The Baby Moses Project](#) offers information and support options for parents who have tried to parent their child but through various circumstances, no longer feel capable of providing for their child.

In addition, put these terms in your search engine to get even more support from your location, including local crisis pregnancy centers.

"This pregnancy was from an affair, and I fear my marriage won't survive if my husband finds out."

Possible Options:

Whatever accountability issue there is surrounding this pregnancy, there are many resources to support you.

Whoever you are afraid of telling, there are professionals in your community ready to support you.

Crisis Pregnancy Centers may provide tips for your situation, as well as referrals to applicable sources.

Marriage counselors are available in every community, through independent listings, bookstore sections on marriage crises or through churches.

"I am young. I have my whole life ahead of me."

Possible Options:

Two things are important to know regarding making a decision to electively abort because you are young. One is that, there are many resources that serve to support you carrying your baby to term while assisting with finishing school and gaining employment. Second, it is important to know that elective abortion has serious long term consequences, and elective abortion performed on young women poses serious, *additional* risks (teenbreak.com).

You can call 1.800.395.4357

Text "TEEN" to 95495

24/7 online chat: option line

In addition, put these terms in your search engine to get even more support from your location.

"I can't afford to take care of this baby."

Possible Options:

Child Support

Government Assistance Programs

Local programs for single parents/low income

Credit card debt support

Mortgage/financial help

SPAOA

Continuing education financial support

In addition, put these terms in your search engine to get even more support from your location.

"I won't have a place to live if I keep this baby."

Possible Options:

Housing Assistance

SPAOA

HUD Housing / HUD.org

Apartments with special programs for single mothers

Pregnancy/mother shelters

Battered women shelters

Au Pair (pronounced "we pair")

In addition, put these terms in your search engine to get even more support from your location.

"My personal safety is in danger if I keep this baby."

Possible Options:

Elective abortion will not inherently increase your safety. If you are in an unsafe situation, it will continue to be unsafe whether you decide on elective abortion or not. You need to get into a safe situation, and there are many resources and places that serve to provide your safety, whichever decision you make regarding elective abortion.

Restraining orders/Ex Parte orders

Pregnancy/mother shelters

Battered and abused women shelters

In addition, put these terms in your search engine to get even more support from your location.

"Selective Reduction: I cannot parent all of these multiples."

Possible Options:

In a culture that has a shortsighted and lofty, almost magical idealism about the splendor of raising multiples, the truth is, raising multiples is enormously challenging. Coupled with the news that any of the multiples might be facing gestational or chromosomal abnormalities, a mother pregnant with multiples might be faced with the decision of what might be called *multifetal pregnancy reduction* or *selective reduction*.

Many of the same resources on this page might be applied in this situation as well.

Our multiples entry page links to practical information for such experiences as twinless twins, which also can be applied in this situation.

Multifetal Pregnancy Reduction, written by Jumelle

Embracing Laura

"The baby has something wrong with him."

Possible Options:

It is extremely important to get a second opinion, from a different hospital, before you make a decision regarding the duration of life in-utero.

Learn what the process of carrying to term is like.

Special Needs Adoption

There are resources that support mothers who are carrying to term babies with all kinds of diagnoses:

Alexandra's House offers, among other things, prenatal and postnatal housing

Madison's Foundation

Congenital Heart Support

String of Pearls

Congenital Diaphragmatic Hernia Support

Congenital Diaphragmatic Hernia Support

Congenital Diaphragmatic Hernia Support

Trisomy Support (13 or 18 or related)

Trisomy Support (13 or 18)

Trisomy 18 support

Trisomy 13 support

Anencephaly support

Prader-Willi Syndrome Support

Spina Bifida Support

Cleft Lip/Palate Support (and related)

Prenatal Partners for Life

Be Not Afraid

Sufficient Grace

Waiting with Love

Beads of Courage

Project Sunshine

NICU support/micropreemie/preemie (scroll to bottom)

Noah's Dad – raising a child with Down's Syndrome from a dad's perspective

These are only a very small number of resources. Please, go slow. You are worthy of support for every single part of this experience you are facing.

In addition, put these terms in your search engine to get even more support from your location.

"No, really. My baby is going to die. It's literally just a matter of when."

Possible Options:

It is extremely important to get a second opinion, from a different hospital, before you make a decision regarding the duration of life in-utero.

Learn what the process of carrying to term is like.

There can be physical, hormonal, emotional, spiritual and psychological benefits to carrying to term. However, carrying to term (or, waiting for spontaneous onset of labor) can also pose very real psychospiritual, social and relational challenges that need to be addressed. Weighing these decisions is an impossible time. What mainstream religious or political agendas don't share openly is that when the death of your baby is entirely unavoidable, as in a diagnosed and confirmed fatal diagnosis, there can be some sense of empowerment in a situation that feels so entirely out of your control, in making such decisions as scheduling the medically assisted birth of your baby, while so doing, forfeiting any or all medicalized life sustaining or death delaying treatment. In a situation such as this, when all circumstances except the date of death and birth are out of your control, the term "elective abortion" may be especially triggering or feel insensitive. The sense of empowerment though, in setting an induction date, can be ongoing, or, it can be fleeting and be met with long term regret. Each member of your care team should be aware and extremely honoring to this truth. "Making a decision and sticking with it" isn't really a reasonable expectation. More in line with the enormity of such a time is to give yourself permission to experience your feelings, and to treat yourself with love. None of this is easy. In any and all of your decisions, go slow. It may feel impossible to go slow, but you can, and prepare your resources for your journey ahead.

"My doctor told me I could die if I don't terminate the pregnancy."

Possible Options:

Like all diagnosis situations, getting a second opinion is always in your best interest.

If your baby has a fatal condition, and waiting for the baby to die naturally poses danger to your own life, here is information particular to your unique situation.

We also have support and resources for children and loved ones when there has been Maternal Death.

Post Elective Abortion

You have Dignity, Worth, and Love

If you have come to this site and have faced elective abortion at any time in the past, seeing the many different perspectives and alternatives, can re-open your wounds and place that heavy burden of guilt on your heart all over again. Grief after elective abortion can look different for each mother. In your grief, you might experience any feelings that are universal to bereaved mothers, such as longing, sadness, or anger. You might also experience feelings of relief, or even feelings of *guilt* at feeling relief. Still other mothers believe that the feelings of regret or shame they may experience are deserved, as if enduring a life of humiliation and comdemnation allows them to bear pain they wanted to protect their children from. These are all complex emotions, and each of them deserve to be looked at lovingly, with a goal of holistic healing. Please know that *you are not alone*, and that there are resources to help you heal, from immediately postpartum, to the lifelong healing journey ahead. Stillbirthday is designed to bring light into the chasm. We are all in this together.

I am Sorry

In some situations, a mother who has decided upon elective abortion may not identify this decision with a "loss". You may not feel a baby died. Your own personal convictions may be that your situation was the "potential" for life, or, that your baby may return to you in a future pregnancy. Into these beliefs, telling you that I am sorry for your loss may not quite fit. But even still, elective abortion can have a substantial print upon your impression of your body image, your feminine identity and your journey. The flow of grief may bring in the occasional shift of breeze that has new questions or new feelings. All of your experiences and all of your feelings are worthy to be looked at with recognition and love. Whatever situation itself that perhaps wasn't the most fertile ground for alternatives to elective abortion, may have been itself a kind of loss, a situation that may hold pain or grief to you. Incest. An unstable relationship. Pressures that made the decision for you. In a later season in which some of these things may change, once again those breezes may blow past your heart and bring fresh questions and feelings. I am sorry. Because being a woman comes with more responsibility than we are ever taught in high school. Because learning to love ourselves is a higher calling than any religious message credits it for. Because we holders of wombs can rip each other to shreds to substantiate our own merit. I am sorry, because I too do not always get things right. I am sorry that it took such a painful subject for us to be real with one another, even here in a tiny written paragraph. I will not wait any longer to tell you. No matter what, you are loved.

Subsequent Pregnancy

Particularly the first pregnancy after elective abortion, you may face the feelings any mother pregnant after loss may endure. In addition to things like climactic milestones in pregnancy (reaching the point in pregnancy in which a diagnosis was determined in a previous pregnancy, the gestational week of birth, or other important points to you), you may find that there are physical and emotional reactions to this pregnancy. The method of medicalized birth, for example, can bring with it long term consequences, such as scarring or impact on fertility and subsequent miscarriage. Emotionally, the pregnancy or climactic milestones within it may be met with fresh grief, fear, guilt, shame, and you may experience stretches of emotional dystocia in labor (a physical delay prompted in part or entirety by emotional implications). However, the emotional impact of a subsequent pregnancy, birth, and choosing an adoption plan or a parenting-through-rearing plan may bring a particular sense of affirmation, reconciliation, peace, and joy. Any or all of these experiences or reactions can be a healthy part of your journey. The decision you have faced regarding the duration of life in-utero is only one part of your story – an important part, but only one part. You can consider how you might define your experience and the unique ways in which you might approach the multitude of aspects of your journey. Maybe you don't feel comfortable sharing openly that you have faced a decision, but, in a subsequent pregnancy, birth or welcoming, you might want to incorporate "rainbows" – which is a common sign among bereaved mothers who have endured pregnancy and infant loss who have a subsequent pregnancy or living baby. Whatever you decide, is as unique and beautiful as you. Please visit our Getting Pregnant Again resources for mothers pregnant after enduring pregnancy and infant loss.

Healing Resources:

SBD Farewell Celebrations

stories contributed by mothers

1.877.586.4621 (Lumina)

1.866.4.EXHALE

National Memorial for the Unborn

Exhale

Hope After Abortion

Post Abortive Reconciliation

After Abortion.org

Your Backline

Bethesda

Lumina

ARIN (Abortion Recovery InterNational)

Rachel's Vineyard (Q&A, retreats, stories)

Supportive Book Listing

Infant Loss Blog Directory has a listing of medical termination blogs (scroll down on the right)

In recognition of the 40th anniversary of Roe v. Wade, CNN published hundreds of small video clips from mothers who have faced elective abortion.

In addition, put these terms in your search engine to get even more support from your location.

You are also invited to share your story with us.

All Are Welcome Here (Please do not drop your flowers and run. You are loved.)

RECURRENT MISCARRIAGE
OR FERTILITY STRUGGLE

This article contains general information regarding recurrent miscarriage, stillbirth, and fertility information. If you are miscarrying right now, please be taken back to the beginning for immediate miscarriage support.

Enduring multiple losses can pose unique emotional challenges, whether you have surviving children or not, and whether you have surviving children or not, emotional support is extremely important. Having a surviving child or children can make you feel as though your feelings over your losses are perhaps less valuable, and well-meaning friends can inflict unintentional harm as they pry and ask questions about your continued family planning, not knowing you may be enduring such heartbreak. If you do not have surviving children, the journey from grief to healing can seem excruciatingly lonely, hopeless, and as though noone could understand your many feelings, including how to handle family pressures to carry on the family name or legacy, or planning your retirement years without children or grandchildren involved.

Whether a few weeks, or a few years, have passed since your first pregnancy loss, any subsequent losses are usually more emotionally devastating on both the mother and the father, and the intensity of the grief can oftentimes seem magnified.

Following subsequent losses, it can seem as though you may be trying to numb or dull the emotions out.

You may have at one time processed your feelings and felt confident that if you experience another loss, you may be more ready, more in control. Oftentimes, it is one parent who feels this confidence, while the other parent may have doubts or fears about trying again. You may feel guilty or embarrassed for thinking you could try again, or for thinking that you could handle another loss easier. You may feel so angry that you decide to make a definitive decision regarding birth control, or you may feel so panicked that you quickly try again. You may wonder why it is so unfair that you have recurrent losses, and may wonder if you'll ever complete a full pregnancy with a happy, healthy baby. You may feel that after subsequent losses, it is best to be quiet about it, not tell anyone, and try to move on silently.

These feelings are all very common, and you really can work through them positively.

And, you are not alone. Please consider sharing your story with us, so that another mother experiencing recurrent pregnancy loss can learn from you.

There are all kinds of support resources here at stillbirthday, from immediate support through the process of loss, to later, long term support resources.

Here are links to several different ideas and sources of information (outside links) that you might find useful. Please discard any resource that does not find comfort in your heart. This is not a place of imposing anyone's position onto you in your journey, or even of endorsing any resource, but simply of presenting different opportunities for you. It is my deepeset desire that you can find a way, a person, or a place, that you feel comfortable talking about your feelings and getting the support that you need.

Multiple pregnancy loss is devastating, and emotional healing is extremely important. Please, as you grieve, and find your way to healing, be gentle with yourself.

Stillbirthday Additional Links:

threatened miscarriage (and some tips)

facts/stats on pregnancy & infant loss

getting pregnant again

loss after medically assisted conception (or ART)

ending fertility in loss

farewell celebrations

Perspectives from Other Mothers:

The Pregnancy Companion (on fertility, adoption, and more)

My Yellow Brick Road Has Potholes

Operation Heads Up (on fertility options)

Peer Infertility Counselors

Professional Fertility Support / Referrals

Fertile Heart

Fertility LifeLine

Prayers for Conception:

Hannah's Tears

Productive Two Week Wait

Sarah's Laughter

Identifying Primary Infertility:

Resolve

A TIME (Jewish support)

Identifying Secondary Infertility:

Resolve

Important Aspects and Links to Fertility Challenges:

Facts/Stats

Fertility after Cancer

Non-Medical Fertility Support:

Fertile Heart

Our Cultural Keepsakes section might be valuable to you.

As with anything, remember to consult your medical care provider.

Non-Medical Fertility and Healthy Links:

Parenting Begins Before Conception

Birth Art Cafe

Pre-Conception Tea

N0n-Traditional Family Support Resources:

Family Creation Network

Medically Assisted Conception:

Ovulation Induction

Ovarian Drilling

Intrauterine Insemination

Female Surgery: Laparoscopy

Female Surgery: Tubal Sterilization Reversal

Female Surgery: Hydrosalpinx Removal

Male Surgery: Testicular Biopsy

Male Surgery: Testicular Sperm Aspiration (TESA)

Male Surgery: Percutaneus Sperm Aspiration (PESA)

In Vitro Fertilization (IVF)

Embryo Donation and Adoption

Embryo Adoption Awareness

Blastocyst/Embryo Transfer

Traditional Surrogacy / Gestational Surrogacy

Surrogacy Laws by State

"All Things Surrogacy"

Foster/Adoption:

Foster/Adopt State-by-State Directory

Adoption Agency Ratings

Center for Adoption Support and Education

Adoption Questions

Missing Grace Foundation

Adoption Doulas or any of our SBD Doulas

Finding Peace with Childlessness:

Beside the Empty Cradle (website)

Beside the Empty Cradle (book)

NICU GRIEF

We have information specific to difficult and fatal diagnosis, including a large listing of outside resources. Please visit our birth plan that can link you to carrying to term information in addition to these outside links specific to diagnoses.

If your baby has received a diagnosis or is expected to receive care in the NICU, here is a list of resources. Please continue to the end of this article for information about *the reality of NICU grief*.

Information for Your Loved Ones:

NICU/Special Needs & Loved Ones

***Prenatal* Educational & Emotional Support:**

Prenatal Process & Support (both surviving & fatal diagnosis)

Bliss

***Immediate & Long Term* Informational & Practical Support Resources for Surviving Diagnosis:**

Infant Disability Resources by State (this large library collection includes a *long term parenting list of resources*)

NICU Items:

Books & Websites relating to the process of carrying to term with a fatal diagnosis

NICU specific clothing

NICU/micropreemie diapers

NICU photography

NICU Support:

Graham's Foundation

Zoe's New Beginnings

Project Sweet Peas

NICU Research & Information:

Some providers discourage parents from touching extreme preemie babies receiving NICU care. This article can give more information on why that is, and what you may be able to do.

Get Connected:

- Share your story here.
- Join our blogroll and other writings here.
- Faith's Lodge & Stillbirthday Mothers Workshops

Many of these are web links that are added to and updated regularly online, but which can't be used through your text, so please visit www.stillbirthday.com for support.

www.stillbirthday.com

NEONATAL DEATH

When a baby dies in the first 28 days of life, it is technically called a neonatal death.

I personally find technical timeframes like this to be arbitrary in our emotional interpretation of our experiences, and I hardly think the term addresses the enormous amount of feeling we may have. We do at stillbirthday provide support for every technical name, medical label, and timeframe category of parental bereavement, including all of the many names for pregnancy loss, neonatal death, older infancy, and toddlers to teens. Just visit here to learn more.

Some parents know ahead of time that their preborn baby may have a condition "not compatible with life" after birth. While these parents may in some ways prepare for the birth of their baby and try to anticipate the very short time they may have with their baby, the experiences are heartwrenching, agonizing and painful.

For these parents, already having a personalized birth plan may help support them through the process.

Still other parents go on to deliver a healthy child, and without any notice or warning whatsoever, the child dies.

In either case, this website offers a number of supportive services:

- information regarding the process from realization to farewell celebration (including a customized birth plan for no or short expectancy of life, and another to serve families when given extra time, and additional resources for various diagnoses). The PROCESS link is extremely valuable.

- statistics

- information for friends and family on how to best support you

- professionals and volunteers to support you

- local, national, and international long-term support services and resources including books

- farewell celebration ideas

- a place to share your story

- a place to read a story or two from other parents and see their babies photos

- please visit our Love Cupboard for newborn clothing support which may prove useful when given extra time.

BIRTH METHODS
The way baby will be born.

Birth methods include the recommended ways, techniques and tools involved to provide the safest birth experience. Just like medical explanations, these pages are derived from www.stillbirthday.com and are written as to the mother.

METHOTREXATE

Methotrexate is administered to mothers who have been diagnosed with an ectopic pregnancy very early in their pregnancy (generally about 6 weeks and under). It can be given orally, however, it is usually recommended that it be administered by injection, with either one or two injection sites. It is considered a noninvasive procedure and reduces the amount of scarring to your reproductive organs. On rare occasions, this medication may also be administered *after* laparoscopic surgery to prevent any cells from growing that may have been left behind.

The medication will simply tell your baby to stop working.

After the medication is administered, you will probably be allowed to return home, with a follow up appointment a few days to a week later.

Within that time, your baby's efforts to grow will be rested to the point that the baby dies.

You will bleed just as in a natural miscarriage, for at least the first few days.

You can make this birth method more meaningful by incorporating your own birth plan.

How far along are you? Because ectopic pregnancy can be fatal to the mother unless the pregnancy ends as quickly as possible, I will only include very early development links to fetal information (and there is a probability that the development of an ectopic baby may be a little different; still, it can be nice to have a general idea of what your baby's last developments will be).

Your doctor will advise you against using any of the following, as they can interfere with the concentration of medication:

- vitamins containing folic acid (including prenatal vitamins)
- alcohol
- penicillin
- ibuprofen

Your doctor will also cover side effects and warning signs with you, including discussing the potential risks Methotrexate (possibly referred to as chemotherapy) can have on trying to conceive in the near future. Some studies indicate that the medicine from Methotrexate may remain present in your own body's cells for up to 7 months after use; doctors generally recommend waiting at least one ovulation cycle before TTC after Methotrexate to prevent complications in fetal growth in the subsequent pregnancy.

LAPAROSCOPIC BIRTH

Surgery for ectopic pregnancy may either be laparoscopy (explained here) or minilaparotomy. Because ectopic pregnancy can be fatal to the mother unless the pregnancy ends as quickly as possible, I will only include very early development links to fetal information (and there is a probability that the development of an ectopic baby may be a little different; still, it can be nice to have a general idea of what your baby's last developments will be). This surgical birth method may be used if methotrexate was ineffective.

The full medical term for laparoscopic surgery is "Laparascopic Salpingotomy". Laparoscopic surgery is performed under general anesthesia. Your doctor will use a tool called a laparoscope to enter your abdomen through a small incision, deliver the baby, and to repair any affected part of the fallopian tube.

Once the doctor determines the condition of the fallopian tube, if it is not repairable, a "Laparoscopic Salpingectomy" will be performed (a "laparotomy", which is a larger abdominal incision, may be required), which is the partial or the complete removal of the damaged fallopian tube.

You can make this birth method more meaningful by incorporating your own birth plan.

Development:
- 4 weeks
- 5 weeks
- 6 weeks
- 7 weeks
- 8 weeks

"NATURAL" MISCARRIAGE

Natural miscarriage means waiting for the miscarriage to complete on its own. A benefit to miscarrying naturally is knowing for certain that your baby in fact has died (see concerns with D&C). It also allows you to spend time gathering your feelings and processing the transition from experiencing hopes and joy to experiencing loss. A common concern that your medical provider may have about you miscarrying naturally, is is the risk of postpartum hemorrhage. The risk of complications of a natural miscarriage is increased, the older the baby was when he or she died. Generally, studies indicate that approximately 70% of mothers who miscarry naturally do so without unexpected complications. Natural miscarriage is safest if the baby's gestational age is younger than *10 weeks*. If you and your medical provider have both determined that natural miscarriage would be a safe option for you, it is important to know what to expect and how to prepare yourself.

If at any time you fill a maxi pad sooner than a half hour, experience dizziness, tingling in your hands or feet, or a racing heart (or any of these even with light bleeding), you should consult a medical professional immediately.

INDUCTION/AUGMENTATION

Medication can help stimulate labor, and allow you to birth your baby.

These are a few common medications that are used to help deliver miscarried babies, and they may be given separately or in conjunction with each other:

- mifepristone
- misoprostol
- methylergometrine (methergine)

Mifepristone blocks a hormone (progesterone) from completing its pregnancy function of supporting the uterine lining that the baby has been growing in. This will stop your body's efforts of sustaining the pregnancy. In some cases, this will be enough to trigger "permission" to your body to begin expelling the placenta and delivering your baby.

Misoprostol (a prostaglandin) causes your uterus to contract, so that your baby can be delivered. "Cytotec" is one prescription name used, and misoprostol is said to have about an 80-90% effectiveness rate in delivering miscarried babies and completely expelling all of the placenta pieces.

Methergine helps to control excessive bleeding and can cause your uterus to contract, so that your baby can be delivered.

You may be asked to stay at the hospital to deliver your baby, or you may be permitted to deliver your baby at home. This will depend on the age of your baby, and other factors including your hospital's policies. Using labor stimulating medication to help with the delivery of your baby in early pregnancy is generally considered a medically safe approach, one that doesn't have the possible adverse side effects as more medically involved births. In rare instances, medication does not deliver the entire placenta, and more medically assisted support (D&C) may be needed to help completely deliver the placenta.

When using a labor stimulant to help in the delivery of a very young baby, you should expect to see a heavier blood discharge than your menstrual period, and possibly small tissue-like pieces of uterine lining. Your baby's placenta, as it detaches from your uterine wall, is very soft and will most likely break into smaller pieces. By the eighth week of pregnancy, the placenta is about the size of a peach, and by the twelfth week it's about the size of a pear, and so the pieces as it is delivered may roughly be the size of grapes.

Your doctor will discuss with you the side effects and warning signs to look out for when taking induction medication, including fever, too much bleeding (hemorrhage), and the amount of time it should take to complete the entire process.

Generally, you will probably be cautioned that filling a regular-absorbancy maxi pad sooner than one hour, at any time, is cause of concern; immediately postpartum (that is, right after the baby is born), generally speaking you should not fill a regular-absorbancy maxi pad sooner than a half-hour in the first hour (so, you can go through 2 pads in the first hour postpartum), as it is common to experience some increased bleeding at the actual time of delivery.

Besides medication to help stimulate labor, other options to assist in the dilation of your cervix may include **seaweed laminaria** or the use of a **Foley catheter**. The Foley catheter (sometimes called Foley ball or bulb) will manually dilate your cervix; this is not a medication but is instead a tool/instrument. Your doctor will insert the Foley into your vagina and the process can be uncomfortable but should resemble a vaginal exam. The ball has a small tube at the end of it. After the ball is in place, the doctor will fill up the ball like a balloon. The sensations from the Foley vary to feeling bloated, crampy, to a feeling of having tetanic (constant) contractions. As you dilate large enough, the Foley will fall out. Each of these options can help dilate your cervix to approximately 3 or 4 centimeters, which should be enough for early pregnancy loss. Pregnancy losses that occur later in pregnancy may be supplemented by the use of Pitocin to continue to dilate the cervix for birth.

Your doctor will discuss these options with you according to your unique situation.

If at any time you fill a maxi pad sooner than a half hour, experience dizziness, tingling in your hands or feet, or a racing heart (or any of these even with light bleeding), you should consult a medical professional immediately.

If you are hoping to be able to find and identify your baby, the chances are increased if you have a general understanding of what to expect to find. The following links will take you to information on the stages of development and the size of the baby.

LEVELS OF AUGMENTATION

There are various ways to help facilitate some change in the progress of labor. Many are listed here, in order from least interventive ("natural") to more interventive ("medical"). Please know that many "natural" techniques are not scientifically proven and/or their effectiveness may be in conjunction with dangerous side effects. Please discuss all "natural" options with your care provider (OB or midwife), whether or not your doula is versed on the topic or not, including exactly how to prepare or present the option. We also note in our early at-home birth plan, that it is possible to experience what we refer to here at stillbirthday as "early pregnancy prodromal labor" – your labor may or may not start and stop, unexpectedly. It is also, enormously important for you to know, for your emotional well being, that even if a "natural" option *might* help in the augmentation of labor, *this does not mean that it caused your loss.* These options are listed here because it has been noted by other mothers, that *once the birthing process has already begun*, these options have been reported by them as being in some way helpful.

Please utilize any of the many emotional support resources we have available at stillbirthday.

External
- walking, lunging, singing, praying/meditating (entering into a safe physical place to do so), relaxing, car ride, oxytocin release (doula can support), massage, effleurage, brushing teeth, hydrotherapy, various "yoga" type positions (doula can support), chiropractic care, herbal bath: yarrow, sage, oregano and nettle.
- stillbirthday has a proprietary collection of healing essential oils, but *shipment times need to be considered.*

External – More Intensive
- nipple stimulation, accupressure/puncture

Internal
- raspberry leaf tea, Lady's Mantle, wine of ergot (spurred rye), eggplant parmesan, oregano, pineapples, spicy foods, "labor cookies", intercourse, coffee or other stimulants
- Spatone, chlorophyll, Floradix, hemoplex, spirulina, alfalfa, red clover or nettle can help restore iron drained through blood loss.
- deep reflection into possibilities of emotional dystocia: prayer, meditation, reflection, permission to heal

Internal – More Intensive
- cohoshes, primrose, fresh parsley, castor oil/enema, cotton root bark, angelica, pennyroyal (please see this external article regarding herbal augmentation) , vodka (some believe that any alcohol, however, can actually stall labor. Again, all of these *need* to be discussed with your provider.)

Medical
- vaginal exams, stripping membranes, cervical ripening agents (Misoprostil), Foley bulb (see Artificial Induction birth method for information on Misoprostil, Foley and other augmentation options)

Medical – More Intensive
- Cytotec, Pitocin, forceps/vacuum/episiotomy, or planned or emergency Cesarean Birth(see Full Term Birth Plan for information on these options)

EARLY TO MID PREGNANCY MEDICALLY ASSISTED BIRTH

D&C AND D&E

If your doctor has recommended a D&E to help deliver your baby, the very first thing to consider is changing the perspective you may have about this approach.

Many mothers have very strong objections to having a D&E performed because of the comparison to an elective abortion.

A D&E is a way to medically assist in the delivery of a baby. The medical operation is the same if the baby is alive or not. But, the operation itself is not abortion. It is a medical way to assist in the delivery of your baby. If this method is needed, perhaps it might be more healing for you to consider it more of a "**vaginal Cesarean**", in that the doctor is going to manually assist in the delivery of your tiny baby.

Another thing you may consider, is that some women recall feeling doubt or uncertainty that their child had in fact died prior to the D&E. This doubt is part of the grieving process, and is normal. But it can be terribly difficult to move past any feelings of doubt or uncertainty *after* the D&E has been performed. For this reason, I strongly suggest utilizing any ultrasound or doppler device that you can prior to the D&E. Perhaps contact a local *crisis pregnancy center* to see if they offer free ultrasounds. This extra step can provide you with the certainty you need in knowing that you are not "electively aborting" your baby. Remember, a D&E does *not* mean elective abortion.

The third thing to consider, is asking your provider if artificial induction may be a simpler, safer way to deliver your baby. Sometimes, a doctor will plan for a D&E (or a D&C, which is a different birth method that may also be an option to ask about) simply because it can be easier on you than trying to really navigate different approaches. Even if your doctor has recommended a D&E, it might be a good idea to just mention the option of artificial induction, and allow your provider to discuss your options with you so that you can have the safest delivery of your baby possible.

Now, with all of that said, a D&E (sometimes mistakenly called a DNE) is a method of delivery, used most often in *inevitable* or *missed* miscarriages, or for miscarriages that occur later in the second trimester, after your baby's bones have begun to harden (approximately at 16 weeks or older). It may also be used if a miscarriage had not completed naturally (any placenta fragments remain in the uterus). It is a combination of the D&C birth method, with additional delivery tools used, such as forceps, to help deliver your baby. We include additional information regarding this in our birth plan, where you might consider what questions or options you may have and create a dialogue with your trusted care provider about ways to learn the gender of your baby, physical characteristics, or anything else that might be of emotional value to you.

You may be given an antibiotic and/or pain medication, and physical recovery may include spotting for several days. Your birth plan for this method will include additional information. Generally, it is best to not plan on conceiving again until after you have had the first subsequent menstrual cycle, to ensure that your uterus is completely clear; waiting at least a week to introduce anything into your vagina (tampons, intercourse) is also recommended. Your provider will discuss these things with you.

You can make this birth method more meaningful by incorporating your own birth plan.

ENCOURAGEMENT FOR BIRTH

These quotes and verses serve to bring encouragement to you *as you prepare for the birth of your baby.* Because pregnancy loss is still birth, these affirmations and encouragements are borrowed from childbirth websites (sources at end) and in fact are more fitting here than anywhere else.

As for you, be strong and courageous, for your work will be rewarded. ~ 2 Chronicles 15:7

"If I don't know my options, I don't have any." ~ Diana Korte

God arms me with strength, and he makes my way perfect. ~ Psalm 18:32

"There is a secret in our culture, and it's not that birth is painful. It's that women are strong." ~ Laura Stavoe Harm

The Lord will fight for you… ~Exodus 14:14a

"It seems that many health professionals involved in antenatal care have not realized that one of their roles should be to *protect the emotional state of pregnant women.*" ~Michel Odent, M.D.

God is our refuge and strength, an ever present help in time of trouble. ~ Psalm 46:1

"The effort to separate the physical experience of childbirth from the mental, emotional and spiritual aspects of this event has served to disempower and violate women." ~Mary Rucklos Hampton

The Lord your God is with you wherever you go. ~Joshua 1:9

"Fear can be overcome only by Faith." ~Grantly Dick-Read, M.D.

Though he brings grief, he will show compassion, so great is his unfailing love. ~Lamentations 3:44

Verses borrowed from: Scriptures for Childbirth
Quotes borrowed from: Birth Without Fear

BIRTH & BEREAVEMENT QUOTES

I would not undo his existence just to undo my pain. ~Stillbirthday Mother

Every baby is born. ~Cathy Gordon, CNM

Miscarriages are labor, miscarriages are birth. To consider them less dishonors the woman whose womb has held life, however briefly. ~ Kathryn Miller Ridiman

Sometimes the heart sees what is invisible to the eye. ~ H. Jackson Brown, Jr.

The love and bond between a mother and her child begins the very moment she knows they are on their way to her. ~ Vicki Reece

Waiting is painful. Forgetting is painful. But not knowing which to do is the worse kind of suffering. ~ Paulo Coelho

Hope is important because it can make the present moment less difficult to bear. If we believe that tomorrow will be better, we can bear a hardship today.
~ Thich Nhat Hanh

A very small degree of hope is sufficient to cause the birth of love. ~ Stendhal

I honor you. {I DO}ula. ~stillbirthday doula

A pregnancy loss is still a birthday.

MY WORDS

07.
BIRTH PREPARATION
"BIRTH PLANS"

EARLY PREGNANCY HOME BIRTH

Things to know:

- You should not miscarry your baby at home alone.

Helpful tips:

- Check out our listing of local professionals and volunteers willing to support you through the process
- Consider special farewell words or music.
- Also include a personalized farewell celebration.
- Ask for your ultrasound photos, if any, or visit a local Crisis Pregnancy Center that performs ultrasounds, and ask if you can have one last photo of your baby.
- If your baby still has a heartbeat, consider using your cell phone or other recordable device, and record the doppler's sounds of your baby's heartbeat. You can then add this to a Build-A-Bear as a momento.
- More momento and special ideas are listed in the birth plan.
- If after the birth, you experience pain, fever, bleeding that fills a pad sooner than an hour, clotting, or a foul odor, please see your care provider immediately. Please view the article on postpartum hemorrhage.
- Our birth education section has additional information that may prove useful to you, including our Levels of Augmentation article that provides ways of naturally augmenting/speeding up the labor process.
- Please visit our link on general postpartum health (your emotional and physical health after delivery).

How far along are you? Do you know what to expect to possibly see? You are invited to view photos shared by other mothers.

www.stillbirthday.com

For babies about 10-19 gestational weeks

Things to Have

Labor

__support person!

__phone (to call 911 if necessary)

__heavy maxi pads (no tampons)

__camera

__plenty of water to stay hydrated

__music and other soothing birth items and options, like massage, affirmations

__do not use a douche or enema to help labor progress

__several large old towels to catch blood in the birth space, especially around toilet

__ small fish net (or plastic bowl, colander, ladle or cheesecloth – you can rest the colander inside the toilet) to help screen or scoop from toilet

__latex gloves (dish or medical gloves) to help scoop from toilet

The Welcoming

__large sheet of tinfoil (or plastic wrap or wax paper) as a stable place to view your baby after birth

__saline (contact solution) to use with clear cup

__clear shot glass or small vase (with saline solution: this helps restore your baby's fullness and can magnify his or her shape so you can see him or her more clearly)

__tweezers or toothpicks to help move fragmented pieces of placenta or sac without sticking and causing unnecessary ripping/sticking

Preparing for The Farewell

__if you are planning on bringing everything that you deliver to the hospital, including as much of the placenta as you can, you will need a large, gallon sized ziplock baggie (and a non-see through grocery sack or bag to place that in)

__special jewelry box or other special box for a coffin for your baby to be placed in

__a small square of pretty gift tissue with a little note that you can flush, or incorporating water in another way, particularly if flushing is inevitable

__be prepared for a possible ER visit

Things to do Before the Birth (while laboring)

__set up your bathroom and/or another room as the birth space. Fold edges of foil to make a large tray, and place this on your counter.

__call friends and family for support.

Things to Expect

__Sometimes bleeding will begin, and then completely stop (for hours or even days) before resuming.

__bleeding should not fill a heavy maxi pad sooner than one hour at any time during the labor.

__the placenta is between the size of a pear to a grapefruit, and will probably be expelled in grape sized pieces.

__very small, fleshy, flaky pieces of discharge are probably pieces of your uterine lining.

__every time you use the restroom, once bleeding has begun, you may expel pieces of placenta.

__it is easier to retrieve everything that is being expelled, to look through and identify your baby, if you hold the small fish net or colander underneath your vagina in the toilet bowl, than it is to allow everything to first be caught in the toilet and attempt to retrieve it after (because everything may be slippery)

__labor will likely peak right before the birth of your baby, at which time, for the first hour postpartum, bleeding may increase, but you should not fill a heavy maxi pad sooner than a half hour, during the first hour (after the first hour, bleeding should begin to taper off).

__know that your baby may not be born intact. He or she may physically be very unrecognizable.

__if you baby is born in his or her amniotic sac, he or she may appear to look very similar to the pieces of expelled placenta.

__when your baby is born, place him or her on the foil tray you have set up on your bathroom counter. Using the tweezers and foil creates a place you can gently pull back some of the additional sac fragments to simply look upon the physical form of your baby. Because physical changes happen rapidly, placing your baby into the clear jar of saline water can help draw out the fullness of his form again and continue to preserve him. You'll need to change this water at least every 4 hours if you choose to keep him in here longer.

__don't use toilet paper or Q tips to dry baby, as it may stick and pull at your baby's delicate skin. Instead, use tweezers, a toothpick, or your finger, and very gently move your baby away from the small puddle of blood, until he or she is more dry. Know that your baby will lose his shape very quickly after birth.

__Utilize all of the special plans you have, including saving mementos, holding your baby.

__name your baby, take photographs

__when you are ready, place your baby in the small Tupperware container and then in the special box.

__invite a spiritual advisor/leader and friends and family to join you after the baby is born (please consider though, that they may not choose to see your baby). See the "Professionals/Volunteers" link at stillbirthday.com for additional services to consider.

After the Birth

If you leave to the ER

__bring a fresh change of clothes with you.

__Have the photo you brought placed with your baby.

__Ask if baby can be swaddled in the blanket you brought (or just leave the blanket there)

__ask if you will be able to take your baby home with you, or if you can have your baby returned to you after any genetic testing is done.

At Home

__Have someone planning on spending the night with you. Perhaps consider having a friend spend the night with you, so that your husband can go home, prepare the house, and rest.

__You will still have lochia (the remaining blood from inside the uterus, which may be shed for the next 1-3 weeks).

__Watch for signs of postpartum depression (PPD) or secondary vaginitus.

__Be easy on yourself, your body, and on your recovery.

__Talk to your trusted spiritual advisors, your husband, and trusted mentors and friends about all of your feelings.

__*Visit stillbirthday.com for "Farewell Celebrations" and for "Long Term Support" resources.

Babies about 4-10 gestational weeks

Things to Have

__The same supplies as listed above

Things to Expect

__labor (bleeding) should begin within two weeks of the death of your baby, but could take longer. Natural induction could include drinking raspberry tea.

__it will be very unlikely that you will be able to identify or retrieve your very tiny baby (flushing is very likely inevitable)

__name your baby

__include a trusted spiritual advisor and friends and family if you wish. See the "Professionals/Volunteers" link at stillbirthday.com for additional services to consider.

After the Birth

If you leave to the ER

__bring a fresh change of clothes with you.

__Have a photo you brought placed with your baby.

__Have a blanket or other special item left with your baby.

__ask if you will be able to take your baby home with you, or if you can have your baby returned to you after any genetic testing is done.

__bring a teddy bear or other item that you can hold on the car ride home.

At Home

__Have someone planning on spending the night with you. Perhaps consider having a friend spend the night with you, so that your husband can go home, prepare the house, and rest.

__You will still have lochia (the remaining blood from inside the uterus, which may be shed for the next 1-3 weeks).

__Watch for signs of postpartum depression (PPD) or secondary vaginitus.

__Be easy on yourself, your body, and on your recovery.

__Incorporate your spiritual beliefs, your husband, and trusted mentors and friends about all of your feelings.

__*Visit stillbirthday.com for "Farewell Celebrations" and for "Long Term Support" resources.

EARLY PREGNANCY OPERATIVE BIRTH

This plan is specific to early pregnancy (under 20 weeks) medicalized, operative birth.
Note that different aspects of the delivery will be different for the different gestational ages.

Birth in hospital: you may be placed under general anesthesia, or sedation, and after the birth, you will stay in recovery for a few hours, when you will be discharged.

Birth at office: the doctor may administer local anesthesia, and your discharge will be in less than an hour (like a pelvic exam).

Please visit the previous chapter to become familiar with the ways in which stillbirthday offers a compassionate explanation and definition for the experience of a medically assisted birth in early or mid pregnancy.

During Birth

What to Bring

__camera
__someone to support you (to wait in waiting room, and to drive you home)
__additional support people can include a friend or chaplain
__photo of you and your husband to keep with baby
__Clinging Cross or something special to hold
__scented eye mask to wear during the birth
__*additional special items: two teddy bears or blankets (one to leave with your baby, and one to take home)
__Music and player (headphones) or battery operated personal fan, if permitted (to muffle the sounds of the surgical delivery)
__Wear your favorite scented lotion or perfume
__If you husband is your support person, have him wear his cologne, aftershave, deodorant, or other smell you prefer
__any ultrasound pictures you may have, favorite scriptures, inspirational quotes or affirmations, that you can read in the waiting room
__letters or cards written from other family and friends that you may have, to be read in waiting room
__pictures drawn by older siblings posted in room (and left with baby)
__incorporation of spiritual beliefs

The Welcoming

During this stage of pregnancy, you may likely be discouraged from seeing your baby. Your baby may not be delivered completely intact physically. If you ask your doctor during the time of the birth, you may be allowed to have your baby's physical form returned to you after their analysis/autopsy of the baby is complete. If you are permitted to have your baby returned to you, a representative of the hospital will likely call you within two weeks of the birth for you to come and receive your baby. He or she will likely be placed in a small container. Please know that your baby's physical form is not going to be intact, and this may be extremely upsetting for you to see. Please consider not opening the container.

Your doctor may also offer suggestions for physical pain relief, including medicinal options. You might also inquire of prescription of estrogen and progesterone treatments, as this has been theorized to reduce the incidence of intrauterine adhesions, therefore possibly preventing future additional fertility challenges as a result of the birth method needed for this pregnancy.

After the Birth

- Have the photo you brought placed with your baby.
- Have the blanket you brought placed with the baby (just leave these items in the room if you like).
- Name your baby
- *See the "Professionals/Volunteers" link at stillbirthday.com for additional services to consider.
- Perhaps consider having a friend spend the night with you.
- You will still have lochia (the remaining blood from inside the uterus, for about a week or less).
- Watch for signs of postpartum depression (PPD) or secondary vaginitus.
- Watch for warning signs including fever, pain, filling a maxi pad sooner than an hour (bleeding after a medically assisted birth should be minimal), clotting, or a foul odor. Please contact your provider immediately if you experience any of these signs.Consult with your OB about TTC. Most will recommend waiting at least 6 weeks, just as in a full term delivery. We have information here regarding TTC (trying to conceive) and getting pregnant again.
- Be easy on yourself, your body, and on your recovery.
- Talk to your trusted spiritual advisor, your husband, and trusted mentors and friends about all of your feelings.
- *Visit stillbirthday.com for "Farewell Celebrations" and for "Long Term Support" resources.

Have at Home After Birth

__people ready to help!
__maxi pads (for lochia, you may have postpartum bleeding for about a week)

STILL BIRTH

This plan is specific to a 31+ week delivery, in which you may be required to stay overnight. You may not be required to stay overnight. Ask your doctor for more information.

Things to Know:

- Because the first plan covers 2 different birth methods, specifics to each particular birth method will be noted.
- Cesarean has its own birth plan because it is so in-depth. You might consider printing both plans, in case your birth turns into an emergency Cesarean.
- This plan is appropriate for pregnancies about 31 weeks to 40 weeks or more.
- These plans do not include specific options you may wish to include if your baby may survive past birth, including possible resuscitation, ventilator use, medications and additional testing. You should consider including these things if there is a chance of your baby surviving for any additional time past delivery.
- If your baby is expected to receive care in the NICU, here is a listing of NICU specific resources and information.
- Some providers discourage parents from touching preemie babies receiving NICU care. This article can give more information on why that is, and what you may be able to do. The NICU experience alone can promote parents grief. Please see our article on Identifying Grief to find information and support regarding grief but also the correlation between the NICU experience and grief/depression/PTSD.
- Within the first 24 hours after your baby has died, there may be an opportunity for you to decide on organ or tissue donation. Please discuss this in advance with your spouse and with your medical professional. Purposeful Gift is an organization founded by an SBD trained doula. You can also learn more by Googling "donor network (your state)", finding your local OPO, or contacting your local organ donation center. Cord blood information can help you determine the likelihood of your donating your baby's cord blood. Here is information specifically for organ donation from an anencephalic baby. Any of these things will depend on a number of factors unique to your situation.
- Get more birth education and learn what to expect during labor, here.
- Please visit our link on general postpartum health (your emotional and physical health after delivery).

Helpful Tips:

- Check out our listing of local professionals and volunteers willing to support you through the process
- Learn about the special way to give a stillborn baby a bath.
- consider hand or feet molds of your baby
- consider inkless prints: fingerprints/handprints/footprints of your baby
- Your body is likely to produce breastmilk after the birth of your baby. Please learn about post loss lactation. This link discusses breastmilk donation in particular.
- If your state doesn't offer a birth certificate for stillbirth, consider printing off our unofficial birth certificate (found at the Farewell Celebrations link).
- Consider special farewell words or music.
- Also include a personalized farewell celebration.
- Ask for your ultrasound photos, or visit a local Crisis Pregnancy Center that performs ultrasounds, and ask if you can have one last photo of your baby.
- Prior to birth, if your baby still has a heartbeat, consider using your cell phone or other recordable device, and record the doppler's sounds of your baby's heartbeat. You can then add this to a Build-A-Bear as a momento. Alternatively, you can purchase a beautiful Angel Heartbeat Bear, which has everything included.
- Prior to birth, consider having a belly cast done as a momento.
- Prior to birth, consult with your doctor and with the funeral home that you select, to see if special considerations

can be made, such as, you leaving the hospital with your baby, to take to the funeral home.
- ☐ More momento and special ideas are listed in the birth plan.

Have an idea of what your baby may look like. You can visit stillbirthday for photos of babies shared by mothers.

What to Pack

__ camera, stillbirthday.com lists professional photographers at the "professionals/volunteers" page.
__photo of you and your husband to keep with baby
__Clinging Cross or something special to hold
__*additional special items: two teddy bears or blankets (one to leave with your baby, and one to take home), mold for baby's hands or feet
__Music and player
__Favorite candle (in glass jar, for warmer)
__Personal fan
__Several wash cloths, for hot or cold compresses (optional-hospitals have plenty)
__Thermos of hot water
__Massage tools: rice packs, rolling pin, paint roller, oil
__Unscented and scented lotion
__Birth ball
__Pillows (1 or 2) and colored cases
__Change of clothes for labor partner
__Snacks for labor partner
__Gum or mints for labor partner!
__Husband's cologne, aftershave, deodorant, or other smell preferred by the mother (he'll wear it)
__Snacks for you: light snacking during birth, orange juice postpartum
__Suckers or other hard candy
__Lip balm
__Cell phone or calling card
__Loose change for phone or snacks
__Phone list for support people to join you for hospital visitation
__Ultrasound pictures, favorite scriptures
__*baby's outfit (for visitation through to final farewell/burial)
__Toiletries: contact case, shampoo, toothbrush, deodorant, etc.
__Night gown or robe (might get soiled)
__Going home outfit for mom (2nd trimester clothes)

Have at Home

__people ready to help!
__maxi pads (for lochia)
__nursing pads (and cabbage, sage tea, and decongestant for expedited weaning, or a hospital grade pump and storage bags/bottles for milk donation) There is more in-depth information regarding post-loss lactation, and ways to help dry quickly or to pump for donation, at stillbirthday, available on the same page that you printed this birth plan.

About the Birth

NOTE: While it can be safe to deliver a very early miscarried baby at home, with precautions such as those listed in the at-home miscarriage birth plan, delivering a stillborn baby at home can come with some complications. If you are adjusting this plan to deliver your stillborn baby at home, please first consult your local police department to make sure that you are in compliance with your state laws regarding at-home stillbirth. Please make sure that you have a professional midwife to support you, particularly one with stillbirth experience. Please know that there can be medical complications in a stillbirth delivery, just as in a "happy" birth. Infection, postpartum hemorrhage, and other medical concerns should be prepared for. You should not deliver your stillborn baby at home alone. The remaining of this plan will pertain to hospital stillbirth delivery.

Natural Options/Information

- IV, with option of Heparin Lock instead
- Blood pressure cuff
- Possible electronic fetal monitoring
- No food or drink
- Possible limited natural induction/augmentation and positions, because of risk of placenta pulling from uterus and causing internal bleeding
- Hands and knees on ball or on bed can be very helpful
- Left Side Lying can be very helpful

Ways of creating a soothing environment for birthing include (but definitely not limited to):

__dimmed lights
__soft music
__massage (scalp, feet, legs, back, even brushing teeth)
__inspirational messages and scriptures written on index cards or spoken aloud
__letters written from extended family and friends who can't attend the birth (read by husband)
__pictures drawn by older siblings posted in room (and left with baby)
__praying
__water therapy (bath until waters rupture, shower, misting spray)
__hot and cold therapy
__intimacy and bonding with husband

Artificial Induction Options/Information

- Possible cervical ripening agents (Cytotec-tablet or Cervidil-similar to a tampon applicator)
- Pitocin (possibly no water breaking)
- Likelihood of Epidural or Narcotic (Stadol, Nubain are examples)

Pitocin Information

- \+ Can start labor
- \+ Can speed up a slowed labor
- \+ Can increase intensity of contractions
- \+ Can stop a postpartum hemorrhage
- \+ Can be regulated and monitored closely
- \+ Can be turned off if necessary
- − Difficult to produce natural progression of contractions
- − Pain from Pitocin is often more difficult to deal with
- − Requires IV and constant monitoring
- − Mom small chance of hyptertensive episodes
- − Mom small chance of titanic contractions
- − Mom small chance of uterine spasm
- − Mom very small chance of coma

Epidural Information

- \+ Catheter into epidural space in spinal column (1st space)
- \+ No need to repeatedly puncture: catheter can re administer or continue dosage
- \+ Given during Active labor (3-7cm)
- \+ Does not alter mom's consciousness
- \+ Can relax mom
- \+ Can help lower blood pressure of a PIH patient with high enough blood platelets
- − Goal of 80% relief, not 100%
- − Completely immobilizes
- − Not administered promptly: same anesthesiologist for entire hospital
- − Chance of longer second stage/ More difficult to push
- − Mom chance of hypotension (drop in blood pressure)
- − Mom chance of itching in face, neck and throat
- − Mom chance of nausea, vomiting
- − Spinal headache healed by patching hole with mom's blood
- − Postpartum headache/backache
- − Uncontrollable shivering
- − Uneven, incomplete or failed pain relief
- − Loss of perineal sensation: inability to push: increase cesarean chance
- − Mom need catheter
- − Mom chance of fever

Narcotic information

- \+ Given IV in Active labor (3-7cm)
- \+ Increases pain tolerance (doesn't eliminate pain, but takes "edge off")
- \+ Can be given ASAP
- − Barbiturate derivative: anticonvulsive and hypnotic properties ("I feel drunk or something.")
- − Wears off/ ACCLIMATION, need for increased dosage
- − Can either increase or decrease labor (unpredictable),

- Can cause mom vomiting
- Can still feel highest peak of intensity, just not building up or let down

Simply ask your medical professional for the most up-to-date information on all options and how to receive comfort in conjunction to their recommendations for your safest experience.

Crowning/Delivery Options:

__I would like the use of a mirror to see the baby's head crowning
__I would like still photography
__I would like to be reminded and encouraged to touch baby's head while crowning
__forceps, vacuum or episiotomy may assist in final delivery of baby
__Umbilical cord may be cut by doctor *Can be cut "long" so that dad may "trim" it later.

These are extremely condensed versions of very basic information about medical options. It is so very important that you create a dialogue with your provider about what your options are, and what if any side effects you may experience, and how to receive support both for the birth and to ease any side effects of any support option.

After the Birth

__*Have the photo you brought placed with your baby.
__*Ask if baby can be swaddled in the blankets you brought.
__*Ask how long your baby can remain with you.
__*Ask if you can give your baby a bath.
__*Ask if your labor room or your postpartum room can be in a quiet location on the floor, where you have less of a chance of hearing other babies, or if you can be transferred to a different floor in the hospital. Transferring to a different floor means that you will not have maternity-specific care, however.
__*If your baby has hair, ask for scissors to cut a lock off.
__*Utilize all of the special plans you have, including saving mementos, holding your baby, capturing baby's smell with a blanket you will take home with you, dressing your baby, naming your baby, taking photographs, and including a pastor and friends and family. See the "Professionals/Volunteers" link at stillbirthday.com for additional services to consider.
__Have someone planning on spending the night with you. Perhaps consider having a friend spend the night with you, so that your husband can go home, prepare the house, and rest.
__You will still have lochia (the remaining blood from inside the uterus, which will be shed for the next 4-6 weeks).
__*You may have breastmilk come in immediately after the birth. You can choose to pump and donate your milk, or go through the process of drying. Drying your milk supply can be done more quickly by drinking sage tea, taking a decongestant, and/or applying frozen or chilled cabbage leaves in your bra (until the soften and warm, and then change out). Expedited weaning takes about a week to complete. Some studies indicate that there may be a link between compounded postpartum depression and early weaning. More information regarding post loss lactation is available at stillbirthday, from the same page you printed this birth plan.
__*Mentally prepare for going home. The first few days at home can be very difficult.
__Watch for signs of postpartum depression (PPD) or secondary vaginitus.
__Be easy on yourself, your body, and on your recovery.
__Talk to your trusted spiritual advisor, your husband, and trusted mentors and friends about all of your feelings.
__*Visit stillbirthday.com for "Farewell Celebrations" and for "Long Term Support" resources.
*are specific to stillbirth

www.stillbirthday.com

CESAREAN BIRTH

This plan is specific to Cesarean birth.

Things to Have:

__same sized clothes (at least one complete outfit)
__high sitting pants (not low cut), no zipper, no belt
__comfortable panties (high waist) may be more comfy than hospital issued panties
__open-bottomed shirts (no elastic around waist)
__scented spa eye sleep mask to cover your eyes in the bright operating room
__slip-on shoes
__Boppy or extra pillows
__ camera, since headphones are rarely permitted in OR, consider pre-recording a favorite song or songs onto your camera to play during prep/before the birth: doula also brings a camera, and stillbirthday.com lists professional photographers at the "professionals/volunteers" page.
__Clinging Cross to bring with you to the O.R.
__*baby's outfit (for visitation through to final farewell/burial)
__*additional special items: two teddy bears or blankets (one to leave with your baby, and one to take home), mold for baby's hands or feet
__there are things that you will not need to bring, that you will see listed at other websites and birth plans, including a carseat

Have at home:

__antacids
__Dannon Activia yogurt (for healthy digestion)
__journal (to remember when to take medications on time)
__high-fiber meals and soups
__people ready to help!
__items listed in this post: natural honey, Goldbond no-talc
__maxi pads (for lochia, and incision)
__nursing pads (and cabbage, sage tea, and decongestant for expedited weaning, or a hospital grade pump and storage bags/bottles for milk donation)

The Process (Prep):

You are not able to eat a certain amount of hours prior (to reduce risk of pneumonia).
The nurse may shave your bikini line (you can do this before labor begins).
You are given an antacid (again, to reduce pneumonia).
IV is set up.
Catheter is set up (it is removed the morning after). *If baby goes to NICU, you may not be able to get up to see her until the catheter is removed.
Blood Pressure, Heart Rate Monitor, and pressure boots (on legs) are in place.
Medicine is administered.

Brought to the Operating Room (possibly before this point). A paper sheet "screen" will block your view of the surgery, and your hands may be tied down to prevent you from spontaneously touching the open area. *Remember to bring your camera, a picture of you and your husband, and a few baby swaddling blankets to O.R.

The Medicine:

There are three ways the medicine adequate for comfortable and safe surgery can be administered.

Epidural: if you were already using this for labor, the nurse can add medicine appropriate for Cesarean to it.
Spinal: most common for Cesarean.
General: sometimes used for emergency Cesarean; no support will be allowed during birth.
You can ask your anesthesiologist about an analgesic that may allow you to be more alert after the baby is born (Duramorph).

Sensations from Medicine:

Instant, warm, tingly feeling in legs and chest (but some women report a "cold" sensation).
Instantly, the feeling of hunger is gone (a good thing!).
Warm feeling may change to cool if your blood pressure drops slightly.
May seem like you can't breathe. If you can talk, you're breathing. Hold your hand over your mouth so you can feel your own breath.

The Process (Birth):

Cut on skin (transverse "bikini cut" is most common)
Separate 6 pack muscle
Cut through peritoneum (a thin membrane)
Move bladder down slightly
Cut in uterus
Deliver baby! Any sensations of pulling or tugging are of the actual birth.
Umbilical cord cut by doctor *Can be cut "long" so that dad may "trim" it later.
Placenta released and removed.
*Baby swaddled, given to dad. Dad: hold baby close to mom's face, and ask the nurse to take pictures of baby, mom, and of you cutting (trimming) the cord.
The birth process can be completed in 5-15 minutes (the entire operation takes approx. 1 hour)
*Keep an extra camera with mom, with easy access to view newborn photos while remaining in Operating Room (may encourage quicker physical recovery).
*Have the photo you brought placed with your baby.
*Ask if baby can be swaddled in the blankets you brought.
*Ask if your baby can remain with you in the OR, or when you will be reunited in a Recovery Room.
*Ask if you can give your baby a bath in the recovery room.
*Ask if your recovery room can be in a quiet location on the floor, where you have less of a chance of hearing other babies, or if you can be transferred to a different floor in the hospital. Transferring to a different floor means that you will not have maternity-specific care, however.
*If your baby has hair, ask for scissors to cut a lock off.

Side Effects:

(common):
- Numbness (you will need to wait for the earliest signs of gaining sensations before moving to "recovery" room, which may be wiggling your toes or slightly lifting a leg—this can take 1-2 hrs)
- Soreness at medicine insertion site
- Ear ringing
- Shivering
- Anxiety
- Constipation
- Difficulty Urinating
- Headache
- Low Blood Pressure
- Nausea
- (other side effects):
- Skin Reaction
- Itching
- Pain at medicine insertion site
- Burning
- Inflammation
- Difficulty Breathing

The Process (Suturing):

("7 Layer Suture"):
- ☐ may heal faster
- ☐ Uterus stitched
- ☐ Bladder returned to place
- ☐ Peritoneum stitched (thin membrane around organs)
- ☐ Loosely stitch 6 pack
- ☐ Carefully stitch fascia (connective tissues of muscle fibers)
- ☐ Loosely stitch fat layer
- ☐ Skin sutures

("3 Layer Suture"):
- ☐ Uterus stitched
- ☐ Bladder returned to place
- ☐ Fascia carefully stitched
- ☐ Skin sutured

After the Birth:

Cesarean location (incision) will be covered in surgical tape.
You may remain in O.R. until you gain earliest sensations (wiggle toes or slightly lift leg) (1-2 hrs)

Your Options (for Support People):

You can have 1 person present with you during the birth (2 people is unlikely, but worth asking). That same person can stay with you in the Operating Room until you are moved to the "recovery" room on the maternity floor, where you will be reunited with your baby.
The person present for the birth can leave the OR after the birth, to go to your "recovery room" and set up your things and prepare the room for you. This person (your husband), and/or your other support person (doula) will most likely not be able to enter the O.R. after the delivery to support you, so you will not be accompanied by a support person again until you are moved to the "recovery" room.

In Recovery Room/Postpartum Room

It's called the same even for vaginal births. It's actually called "LDR" for Labor Delivery Recovery. After a few hours, you may be moved (again!) to a Postpartum room.

*Utilize all of the special plans you have, including saving mementos, holding your baby, capturing baby's smell with a blanket you will take home with you, dressing your baby, naming your baby, taking photographs, and including a pastor and friends and family. See the "Professionals/Volunteers" link at stillbirthday.com for additional services to consider.

Have someone planning on spending the night with you. Perhaps consider having a friend spend the night with you, so that your husband can go home, prepare the house, and rest.

You will still have lochia (the remaining blood from inside the uterus, which will be shed for the next 4-6 weeks).
For comfort, try putting a maxi pad between your underwear and the birth location (incision). Ask your doctor about adding Gold Bond (no talc) powder to the pad to keep the area dry, or Manuka honey on the incision to aid in it staying sealed.

Get propped up with extra pillows, use Boppy if it helps.

You may be prompted to walk sometime between a few hours to 12 hours after the birth.
Your catheter will be removed within the first 12 hours after the birth.

Gentle, careful movement is best. Walk for a few minutes, every few hours of the day for the first few days. This can actually help with the abdominal discomfort. Walk for a few minutes every hour of day after that (with doctor approval).
Get out of bed by first dangling your feet over, then move to a sitting position. Reverse this to get back into bed: sit on the bed first and slide into your pillow, holding the rail for support.

You may not be able to eat until you pass gas. Walking carefully may help this.

You might feel constipated, and may be given a stool softener.

Respiratory therapy may continue for the first couple of days postpartum. Holding your hands or a pillow over your incision area can help support it while you take deep breaths.

Narcotics are usually given for the first 12-24 hours after the delivery. Take them correctly.

Pain medications are given after that. Take them correctly. Pain is easier to manage before it peaks–delaying medication can make it difficult to manage the pain.

Ibuprofin lowers inflammation=better healing and comfort.

*You will have breastmilk come in immediately after the birth. You can choose to pump and donate your milk, or go through the process of weaning. Weaning can be done more quickly by drinking sage tea, taking a decongestant, and/or applying frozen or chilled cabbage leaves in your bra (until the soften and warm, and then change out). Expedited weaning takes about a week to complete. Some studies indicate that there may be a link between compounded postpartum depression and early weaning.

Have husband or a journal to remind you when to take medications.

Rest. Healing happens when you sleep.

It can take 1-2 whole months for complete healing. Don't over-do it.

*Mentally prepare for going home. The first few days at home can be very difficult.

Watch for signs of postpartum depression (PPD) or secondary vaginitus.

Remember to stay connected to your spiritual support system as well.

Sensations (at birth location)

(worse in the first few days):
- Pulling
- Tugging
- Burning
- Aching
- Itching
- Red
- Puffy
- Uterus Cramping (even for vaginal births, as uterus is shrinking)
- Occasional Sharp Pain, in abdomen, chest, or shoulder area (may be from air entering abdomen during birth—a gas relief medicine may be recommended to get the air out)

Warning Signs

- Bleeding at site
- Oozing at site
- Site opening up
- Smelling bad at site
- Persistent pain
- Fever
- Difficulty breathing

Help Yourself Heal

(Massage)
- Find a massage therapist or physical therapist experienced with Cesarean recovery.
- Myofascial release techniques (gentle pressure applied above the affected area (feeling of tugging or bumpy)
- Cross Friction (Encourages proper formation of scar tissue)

(Other)
- Avoid stairs
- don't waste walking (keep things close)
- Lift nothing heavier than a few pounds
- Do NOT drive
- No sex for 6 weeks (same as vaginal birth)
- Your doctor may recommend not TTC for at least 6 months
- Drink water frequently
- Nap often
- Limit visitors
- Move gently, and as recommended (a few minutes every few hours at first)
- Listen to your body. After the first week, you may be able to stretch your body out a bit more, with pelvic tilts, leg lifts and other gentle stretches.
- Ask friends providing meals to prepare soups for easy digestion, or meals high in fiber to help with your intestinal movements.
- Be easy on yourself, your body, and on your recovery.
- Stay connected to your spiritual beliefs, your husband, and trusted mentors and friends about all of your feelings.
- *Visit stillbirthday.com for "Farewell Celebrations" and for "Long Term Support" resources.

www.stillbirthday.com

FATAL DIAGNOSIS

This is an informational article on what to possibly expect to have occur from the time you discover a difficult diagnosis, through the birth, to the farewell celebration that you choose to honor your baby.

1. **The very first consideration to make is in working through your feelings.** You may experience any of these feelings, either immediately, or through the duration of your pregnancy, and these are not in any order. You need to know that other parents have come before you on this overwhelming journey, and they have felt these very same feelings:
- sadness
- anger
- disbelief
- disappointment/resentment
- jealousy of others
- shame
- shock
- acceptance/peace/even joy over your own pregnancy and child

Studies show that this "pre-grief", or "anticipatory grief", grief experienced prior to the actual death of your child, does not substitute the grief that will occur after your child dies. You will likely experience all of these feelings, and more powerfully, in the days, weeks and even years after the birth and death of your baby.
More information regarding grief and emotions can be found at our emotional/spiritual link.

2. **You need to get support around you.** Decide on who will walk this journey with you, and know that in most cases, your loved ones truly want to be a support to you, although they will likely feel ill equiped. They need their own resources and support, too, and it may take you to let them know that, if their questions become overwhelming and take away from the time you need to sort through your own feelings and experiences. Consider including any of the following people, or others:

- your parents and/or in-laws (Nothing Without You was started by a stillbirthday mother, who has resources for parents and for grandparents)
- closest friend(s) and family (guide them to the family/friends link)
- perinatal hospice support in your local area
- Alexandra's House or other prenatal and/or postnatal housing assistance and support
- professionals experienced with your baby's diagnosis in your area (including transferring prenatal care to a different doctor or hospital)
- other supportive professionals and volunteers in your area, like doulas and photographers (pregnancy/birth/farewell – listed at stillbirthday by state)
- bereavement support in your local area (visit the long term support services link)
- pastor
- professional counselor
- specific support groups or resources if this diagnosis indicates likelihood of future infertility, such as Hunter's Syndrome, Mitochondrial Disease, or Spinal Muscular Atrophy
- additional support services such as the cost of ultrasound provided by Sustaining Grace
- other moms who've come before you. You can read stories by clicking on "All Newborns/Diagnosis" in the right sidebar of this site.
- you can decide how you want to tell your loved ones. Starting a blog for your baby is a great way to work through your feelings, have a special online place that honors your baby, as well as allows others to see what's happening without seeming intrusive.

3. **You are still pregnant, with a live child inside you.** Your baby's experience in-utero is not totally conditioned on your perceptions or feelings toward your experience and this journey. However, it is important to come to find ways of celebrating this pregnancy and bonding with your baby now, while you can. Consider any of these things:

- prayer. It releases oxytocin, sending this oxygen-rich love hormone through your bloodstream to be received by your baby.
- connection with your husband, including sexual and non-sexual intimacy and togetherness. Getting a couples massage or retreating to a bed & breakfast weekend getaway in the country is a great idea.
- purchase a Build-A-Bear with personalized audio recording, to bring to an OB appointment with you. Record your baby's heartbeat, to be put in the bear.
- have a pregnancy belly casting done.
- have a Celebrating Pregnancy blessingway (Sacred Circle) with your closest friends.
- sing and talk to your baby, and touch your belly.
- journal, or write letters to your baby.

4. Prepare for the birth while you are pregnant:
- view our birth planning information that includes information on lactation, NICU, and more.
- consult with your OB over your hospital policies regarding infant death. Ask about:
- homebirth or other options
- the care that will be given to your baby. Are you planning on offering comfort care, or palliative, medical care? If your baby will receive intense medical support, investigate the possibility of delivering at your local intensive care children's hospital, to prevent a transfer of care after delivery.
- time you can have with your baby after delivery (any concerns or possible situations that would limit this)
- what to expect your baby to possibly look like (we accept donations from mothers of photos of their babies, so that mothers coming after you can help get an idea of what to possibly expect. Please submit photos to Heidi.Faith@stillbirthday.com and they will be added to the "Gestational Age of Your Baby" tab, after all of the weeks of pregnancy photos.
- visit or call the maternity floor, and ask if there are nurses there with experience with babies with your baby's diagnosis
- rooming-in with your baby, kangaroo care/skin-to-skin bonding, breastfeeding
- ask if shots, ointments, and screening can be delayed or just not performed
- if your baby lives longer than expected and is able to leave the hospital with you, ask ahead of time what to expect in caring for your baby
- if your baby is not expected to live longer than your hospital stay after delivery, ask about making special arrangements to take your baby to the funeral home (if you can do it, or not)

5. Preparing for your baby's death now, while you are still pregnant, is very emotionally difficult, but it may allow you to create specialized plans for your situation.
- consult with different funeral homes, asking them what their experience is in infant death, and what special arrangements they might be able to offer in your specific situation.
- ask if they can arrange for you to bring your baby from the hospital to them.
- if they cannot do this, ask if, when they arrive to the hospital for your baby, if their representative can carry your baby out of the hospital in their arms, just like a live baby.
- see our Farewell Celebrations for additional suggestions.

www.stillbirthday.com

Additional Support:

Books
Waiting with Gabriel
A Gift of Time
Empty Cradle, Broken Heart
More Books
Websites
Diagnosis & Surviving:
Down Syndrome Pregnancy
Medical Dwarfism
Fatal Diagnosis:
Cherishing the Journey
String of Pearls
Birth Plan (from String of Pearls website)
Growing through Affliction (a letter from one mother to you)
Special Needs Adoption
Madison's Foundation
Congenital Heart Support
Congenital Diaphragmatic Hernia Support
Congenital Diaphragmatic Hernia Support
Congenital Diaphragmatic Hernia Support
Trisomy Support (13 or 18 or related)
Trisomy Support (13 or 18)
Trisomy 18 support
Trisomy 13 support
Anencephaly support
Prader-Willi Syndrome Support
Spina Bifida Support
Cleft Lip/Palate Support (and related)
Prenatal Partners for Life
Be Not Afraid
Sufficient Grace
Waiting with Love
Beads of Courage
Project Sunshine
Purposeful Gift
Noah's Dad – raising a Down's Syndrome child from the dad's perspective
NICU support/micropreemie/preemie (scroll to bottom)
In addition, put these terms in your search engine to get even more support from your location.

Fatal Diagnosis Information

Prepare for the birth while you are pregnant:
- view our birth planning information that includes information on lactation, NICU, and more.
- consult with your OB over your hospital policies regarding infant death. Ask about:
- homebirth or other options
- the care that will be given to your baby. Are you planning on offering comfort care, or palliative, medical care? If your baby will receive intense medical support, investigate the possibility of delivering at your local intensive care children's hospital, to prevent a transfer of care after delivery.
- time you can have with your baby after delivery (any concerns or possible situations that would limit this)
- what to expect your baby to possibly look like
- visit or call the maternity floor, and ask if there are nurses there with experience with babies with your baby's diagnosis
- rooming-in with your baby, kangaroo care/skin-to-skin bonding, breastfeeding
- ask if shots, ointments, and screening can be delayed or just not performed
- if your baby lives longer than expected and is able to leave the hospital with you, ask ahead of time what to expect in caring for your baby
- if your baby is not expected to live longer than your hospital stay after delivery, ask about making special arrangements to take your baby to the funeral home (if you can do it, or not)

This plan is specific to your baby being born, and then dying during your hospital stay or shortly after birth. There are additional notes and options given, for a situation in which your baby survives longer than expected and may be discharged from the hospital with you. Whichever outcome you are expecting, it may be best to at least have some information regarding the other possible outcome.

What to Pack

__ camera, stillbirthday.com lists professional photographers at the "professionals/volunteers" page.
__photo of you and your husband to keep with baby
__Clinging Cross or something special to hold
__*additional special items: two teddy bears or blankets (one to leave with your baby, and one to take home), mold for baby's hands or feet
__Music and player
__Favorite candle (in glass jar, for warmer)
__Personal fan
__Several wash cloths, for hot or cold compresses (optional-hospitals have plenty)
__Thermos of hot water
__Massage tools: rice packs, rolling pin, paint roller, oil
__Unscented and scented lotion
__Birth ball
__Pillows (1 or 2) and colored cases
__Change of clothes for labor partner
__Snacks for labor partner
__Gum or mints for labor partner!
__Husband's cologne, aftershave, deodorant, or other smell preferred by the mother (he'll wear it)
__Snacks for you: light snacking during birth, orange juice postpartum
__Suckers or other hard candy
__Lip balm
__Cell phone or calling card
__Loose change for phone or snacks
__Phone list for support people to join you for hospital visitation
__Ultrasound pictures, favorite scriptures
__*baby's outfits (for visitation through to final farewell/burial)
__*several different folding-style hats and gauze for baby with cephalic diagnosis
__*organ and breastmilk donation and other things you may have decided – and the ability to change your mind about any decision at any time
__Toiletries: contact case, shampoo, toothbrush, deodorant, etc.
__Night gown or robe (might get soiled)
__Going home outfit for mom (2nd trimester clothes)
__a carseat, in the event that your baby survives longer than expected and can return home with you

Have at Home

__people ready to help!
__maxi pads (for lochia)
__any equipment that you may need in the event that your baby will survive a short time and be able to come home with you
__nursing pads (and cabbage, sage tea, and decongestant for expedited weaning, or a hospital grade pump and storage bags/bottles for milk donation) There is more in-depth information regarding post-loss lactation, and ways to help dry quickly or to pump for donation, at stillbirthday, available on the same page that you printed this birth plan.

Birth

Natural Options/Information

- IV, with option of Heparin Lock instead
- Blood pressure cuff
- Possible continuous fetal monitoring
- No food or drink
- No standing, because of risk of placenta pulling from uterus and causing internal bleeding
- Hands and knees on ball or on bed
- Left Side Lying

Ways of creating a soothing environment for birthing include (but definitely not limited to):

__dimmed lights
__soft music
__massage (scalp, feet, legs, back, even brushing teeth)
__inspirational messages and scriptures written on index cards or spoken aloud
__letters written from extended family and friends who can't attend the birth (read by husband)
__pictures drawn by older siblings posted in room (and left with baby)
__praying
__water therapy (bath until waters rupture, shower, misting spray)
__hot and cold therapy
__intimacy and bonding with husband

Crowning/Delivery

__I would like the use of a mirror to see the baby crowning (know that your baby's diagnosis may increase the chances of a face-first presentation)
__I would like photography
__I would like to be reminded and encouraged to gently touch baby's head while crowning (you should discuss this with your OB prior to labor)
__forceps, vacuum or episiotomy may assist in final delivery of baby
__Umbilical cord may be cut by doctor *Can be cut "long" so that dad may "trim" it later.

After the Birth

__*Have the photo you brought placed with your baby.
__*Ask if baby can be swaddled in the blankets you brought.
__*Decide if you would like to delay or forfeit all standard medical support after your baby is born and focus on bonding and time together, or if you would like standard medical support for newborns, including Erythromycin in her eyes, Vitamin K injection, bulb suctioning of her nose and mouth to clear the airways, and APGARs.
__*Decide if you want your baby weighed and measured.
__*Decide if you would prefer life saving medical support, including positive pressure ventilation, intubation or chest compressions, or if the focus should be on comfort.
__*Decide if you want pain medication administered to your baby in the event he or she is in pain.
__*Ask how long your baby can remain with you.
__*Ask if you can give your baby a bath.
__*Ask if your labor room or your postpartum room can be in a quiet location on the floor, where you have less of a chance of hearing other babies, or if you can be transferred to a different floor in the hospital. Transferring to a different floor means that you will not have maternity-specific care, however.
__*If your baby has hair, ask for scissors to cut a lock off.
__*Utilize all of the special plans you have, including saving mementos, holding your baby, capturing baby's smell with a blanket you will take home with you, dressing your baby, naming your baby, taking photographs, and including a pastor and friends and family. See the "Professionals/Volunteers" link at stillbirthday.com for additional services to consider.
__Have someone planning on spending the night with you. Perhaps consider having a friend spend the night with you, so that your husband can go home, prepare the house, and rest.
__You will still have lochia (the remaining blood from inside the uterus, which will be shed for the next 4-6 weeks).
__*You will have breastmilk come in immediately after the birth. You can choose to pump and donate your milk, or go through the process of drying. Drying your milk supply can be done more quickly by drinking sage tea, taking a decongestant, and/or applying frozen or chilled cabbage leaves in your bra (until the soften and warm, and then change out). Expedited weaning takes about a week to complete. Some studies indicate that there may be a link between compounded postpartum depression and early weaning. Additional information regarding post loss lactation can be found at stillbirthday, from the same page as this birth plan.
__*Mentally prepare for going home. The first few days at home can be very difficult.
__Watch for signs of postpartum depression (PPD) or secondary vaginitus.
__Remember to pray and ask others for help and for prayer.
__Be easy on yourself, your body, and on your recovery.
__Talk to God, your husband, and trusted mentors and friends about all of your feelings.
__*Visit stillbirthday.com for "Farewell Celebrations" and for "Long Term Support" resources.

WHEN GIVEN EXTRA TIME

The following information is specifically for babies who survive a longer time after birth:

When Given Extra Time

Provide breastmilk: Begin by pumping your milk, just shortly after the birth. Pump on a regular schedule even if you cannot give it to your baby right away (the hospital will help you store it), or even if milk doesn't come in abundantly. For different reasons, you may have a difficult time initially getting your milk to come in. Providing breast milk for your child is the one thing you can do for your baby that no one else can. Your baby may feed with a nasogastric tube, and can receive your breastmilk that way. Your breastmilk may actually provide a sort of "sterilization" to this tubing, because of the sIgA and other proteins present. You might consider introducing a pacifier after each tubal feeding, to allow your baby to associate suckling with being fed. Latching on can be difficult for babies who haven't yet developed the ability to suckle and breathe at the same time. Once baby latches on, he may eat often, but you will need to pump after feedings to empty the breast. You can begin feeding approximately every two-three hours after a good breastfeeding relationship has been established. Ask for help: utilize lactation support and contact the professionals around you for support.

These are tips to help breastfeed your baby, borrowed with permission from a mother whose experience is similar to yours:

- As soon as possible, hold your baby skin-to-skin, also called "kangaroo care".
- Pump as soon as possible, and for 20 minute sessions, every 2 hours; do not reduce this to less than 8 pumping sessions in a 24 hour period.
- When pumping to increase supply, pump for a few minutes after the last drop.
- When pumping to increase supply, consider "cluster" or "power pumping". Cluster pumping is pumping every half hour to hour for several hours. Power pumping is doing as absolutely minimal work but staying in bed and resting and pumping for 2-3 days.
- As soon as possible, let your baby nuzzle your breast.
- Don't overstimulate with rocking while they are trying to nurse.
- Use the crossover hold.
- Weigh your baby before and after a feeding, without changing the diaper. The grams gained are almost exactly equal to CC's of breastmilk.
- Invest in a scale and an SNS for home (and Tommee Tippee breastflow–not drop-ins) . Your NICU nurse may give you an SNS for free. You can use an SNS and a nipple shield at the same time if you need to. Put the tube on your nipple (a little past the nipple on top), and roll on the nipple shield like a condom, give the SNS a squeeze to fill the nipple of the SNS and then latch the baby on.
- Have your baby's tongue checked for tongue-ties and pallet issues.
- Ask about cup feeding.
- Ask about going home with your baby still on the gavage (see the study from Cochrane for more information.)

2. **Bond with his caregivers:** Natalie, the mother of a 25 week baby, said, "Although you can't do a lot with a 25 weeker, it's nice to know how your baby is used to being handled by the nurses and doctors. This way, when you DO take over care, you can maintain consistency for your baby and help him/her to feel safe. In addition, knowing what was going on – in detail – helped me feel like I was getting to know (my daughter's) personality even though I couldn't interact with her the way normal mothers can. Like how much she liked to try to extubate herself, and how much she hated those wipe-down baths."

3. **Talk to your baby**: If you feel silly talking to a baby, read a book. It doesn't have to be a children's book – any will do! If you can't go to the hospital as often as you want, record your voice talking and singing to your baby. The staff can play it when you aren't there.

4. **Hold your baby**: Hold your baby as much as possible, but know that the earlier a baby is born, the more likely they are to be unable to tolerate touch. Touch can be painful or upsetting to the baby, and they show this by dropping their heart rate and oxygen levels. It's very hard, but those are your baby's cues that, just for right now, he wants to be left alone. Just as you would respect a term baby's cues to be left alone to sleep, you need to respect your preemie's cues.

5. **Decorate his room**: Bring in pictures from home – your older children, your pets, the grandparents. Bring in special stuffed animals and colorful blankets to cover the incubator. Make this "new home" as homey as possible.

6. **Leave your scent**: You, your husband, and your older children can sleep with some soft cloth items and leave them for your baby. Large burp cloths and receiving blankets work especially well. You can pump with a burp cloth under your breasts so that any milk that drips can catch on the cloth, and then you can leave the cloth for him. Later, after he's had it for awhile, you can hold it close to smell your baby as you pump; his scent can facilitate a milk "letdown."

7. **Dress your baby**: As soon as the staff gives you permission, bring in his clothes. Don't worry if they don't fit perfectly.

8. **Take pictures**: Put together a little photo album to share with your friends. Your baby is a gift and should be celebrated!

9. **Celebrate your baby**: Find joy in his birth, and other "firsts", like his first bath or the first time he comes off of the vent. Take pictures and enjoy his tiniest, newest milestones.

10. **Pray**: Let the miracle of your child's life stay the priority while managing the conflicting and painful feelings of the experience. Get support, and keep an eye for signs of postpartum depression. Connect with other parents and with your church family and allow others to pray with you and share in the ways God is moving in the life of your family.

HOME STILL BIRTH

Understand your local laws regarding home stillbirth. Different state laws also provide for different regulations regarding stillbirth at home, particularly if there is a chance for survival. If your state laws permit you to have a home stillbirth, also determine if you have legal permission for any unique plans you have, such as burying your baby at a private cemetery. Your local officials can help you navigate your legal decisions.

Determine if homebirth will prevent life-saving or death-delaying medical support available from a hospital. If you know or even suspect that you may deliver a baby with a serious diagnosis but who also has even a slim chance of survival, you may decide to deliver your baby at a hospital, or discuss a transfer after birth with your midwife.

Consider any medical concerns that may impact your own health, including possible hemorrhage, uterine rupture, and infection. Discuss these risks with your midwife and make a plan to manage these.

Keep all diagnostic medical records from your pregnancy, including any ultrasound images that determine the demise of your baby. You will want to have these available at the birth, as your state laws may require you to present them to your local law enforcement official shortly after the delivery.

Work ahead of time with the funeral home of your choice. Learn their policies. Do they require arriving at your home to transport your baby to their facility? Will they permit you to transport your baby to their facility? Is there a timeframe from the time of delivery in which this transportation needs to occur?

Contact your local law enforcement officials at a responsible time after the birth, if this is included in your local laws (it likely is). They will need to see the diagnostic medical documentation that you've kept through your pregnancy, and ensure that you are safe. Please be respectful and comply with their questions.

Your midwife will need to have the official paperwork to submit to your local Vital Statistics office, to submit a request for an official Certificate of Death (this step may or may not be particularly difficult in your state).

To find ways of making your home stillbirth special, please consider viewing the hospital stillbirth plans as they may provide some support for you in your situation. Our birth education also has useful information.
Please visit the Farewell Celebrations section for support after the birth.

Please also consider sharing your story of home stillbirth, and read the stories of home stillbirth from other mothers.

WATER BIRTH

Hydrotherapy is gaining increasing recognition as a homeopathic ingredient in birth planning.

Water can be included in labor and birth in a number of ways:

- showering, allowing the water to splash onto your breasts and down your belly, to help stimulate labor
- showering with your spouse to help increase oxytocin, to help stimulate labor
- foot soak to ease tension and swelling

Waterbirth can take place at home, at a birth center, or in many hospitals. Contrary to its name, waterbirth not only means giving birth to your baby while you are emerged in water, it is also lesser understood to simply mean spending time soaking while in labor, whether or not the actual birth takes place while still emerged in the water.

Related: at home early pregnancy birth   and   at home stillbirth

Additionally, having a warm bath immediately after the birth can be soothing.

So, can a mother giving birth to her beloved miscarried or stillborn baby still enjoy the benefits of a waterbirth?

The answer? It depends on a number of very individualized and important factors, but YES, waterbirth may indeed still be a valid option.

If you have read through our birth planning materials, have consulted with your care provider, and desire to plan a waterbirth of your miscarried or stillborn baby, here are a few things to consider:

Including Epsom Salt at the measured amount directed on the carton can be particularly advantageous, for the following reasons:

- Magnesium Sulfate is an FDA category A (good to know for mothers experiencing a threatened miscarriage).
- Magnesium Sulfate can help reduce the risk of postpartum hemorrhage, a very serious danger which can be heightened for mothers giving birth via natural miscarriage.
- Because hemorrhage is such a very serious and potentially life threatening issue for mothers experiencing pregnancy & infant loss, it is wise for you to consider that most generally during any water birth, blood released into the water can give an alarming appearance. Additionally, when you first stand up from your bath, you should do so carefully. Mothers giving birth in any trimester should never do so alone. Water and blood that has pooled in your vagina can also give an alarming appearance when you emerge from the water. Please be sure to read our information about hemorrhage because it is such a critical aspect of your experience.
- Magnesium Sulfate has been used intravenously to stall preterm labor, but its actual ability to stall labor is inconclusive. In miscarriage labor, it is already possible for labor to start and stop over a timeframe up to weeks. Knowing this is helpful in your decision making.
- Magnesium Sulfate can help fight infection because of its vasodilatation.
- Soaking for 10 minutes at a time, in warm, fresh clean water, is recommended, when using Epsom Salt or not. This also helps to prevent reabsorption of your toxins flushed during the soak.
- When you have high levels of stress, your body can deplete its source of Magnesium Sulfate, resulting in higher amounts of adrenaline production. These higher amounts of adrenaline can add to the already emotionally overwhelming experience of pregnancy and infant loss, and can even pose additional health risks. Soaking in a warm bath with Magnesium Sulfate can counter these dangers.

The saline water of your soak may aid in preserving the very delicate physical form of your miscarried baby. Using a small fish net to remove fragments of your baby's placenta from your bath may be helpful. Please see our at home birth planning for more information.

You might also add essential oils to your bath.

08.
THE WELCOMING:

HOW TO BATHE & PHOTOGRAPH A STILLBORN BABY
IMMEDIATE POSTPARTUM WELLNESS

BATHING A BABY NOT ALIVE

This article works in conjunction to our article that describes what to expect from the appearance of your baby, and the condition of your baby's skin. Please see The Skin of Your Stillborn for additional information.

Even the smallest of babies can benefit from a bath of sorts – babies born before ossification begins (approximately 16 or 17 weeks gestation and younger), can be gently placed in a clear container of saline water, which can allow the parents to hold and bond with their baby without damaging the physical form, and, this water can help restore a visible "fullness" of the physical form. You can visit our early pregnancy at home birth plan for more information.

In early pregnancy, holding the baby's physical form in saline water can resemble the purposes of a bath: bonding and personhood.

Caregivers often are concerned about showing a stillborn baby to the parents, because of the compromised condition of the baby's body. A baby who has been dead in utero for even a short time can have macerated and discolored skin and a misshapen head. Cleansing the skin of the compromised baby often may be viewed as adding more injury because the skin will slip even farther if a wash-cloth is used. The following information gives practical suggestions on how to care for a macerated stillborn infant.

1. Place the baby into a bath basin of warm bath water which has had baby shampoo added (I like to add Serenity essential oil).

2. Squeeze a washcloth with this shampoo water over the baby's body; do not rub.

3. With gloved hands, place baby shampoo in hands and gently glide over the stillborn's body to remove all drainage. Shampoo the hair gently also.

4. Next take the baby out of the shampoo water and discard the bath water. Rinse the soapy water off the baby by placing in a basin of warm water or by holding the baby under a gentle stream of warm running water from the faucet.

5. Take the baby from the rinse water and place on absorbent towels or underpads. Dab with a soft cloth, such as a Chix, to dry the baby – do not rub.

6. Place Vaseline gauze over macerated areas and hold in place with dry gauze wrap.

7. Transparent dressings (i.e. Opsite or Tegaderm) can be used over macerated areas if the skin next to these areas is intact. This type of dressing can be used over a weeping autopsy incision as well.

8. Dry ear canals and nostrils with Q-tips, gently.
9. If nostrils continue to seep fluid, place a small amount of petroleum jelly into each nostril. This will give shape to the nose and prevent further seepage.

10. Choose clothing that opens completely from the front or back. The important thing is to have clothing that promotes the least amount of handling and rubbing of the stillborn's skin. The least amount of handling prevents further skin slippage.

11. Parents appreciate their baby dressed in blue clothing for a boy and pink clothing for a girl. Sometimes only blue or pink blankets may be available; use the appropriate color.

12. Diaper the baby.

13. Use a baby brush or comb to comb the baby's hair. A bow can be placed in a baby girl's hair by placing a small amount of petroleum jelly on the back of the bow to hold the bow in place. Give the comb or brush to the parents for a memento.

14. Snip a lock of hair from the back of the baby's head for the parents' baby book. Be sure this is within the family's culture or belief before providing this memento.

15. If the baby's head is misshapen, find a cap or hat that when tied under the chin makes the baby's face appear more round. Fill in areas of the hat with gauze or cotton balls if more roundness is needed.

16. When taking the stillborn baby to the parents, line the baby blanket with absorbent underpads so any further weeping can be collected in the underpad without saturating through the baby blanket. Spraying the underpads and the blanket with a commercial baby powder freshener gives a pleasant baby scent memory and lasts longer than baby powder.

How to Take Photos of a Stillborn Baby

17. Take pictures of the baby clothed and unclothed in uncluttered backgrounds. Sinks, garbage cans, cleansing equipment do not provide backgrounds for memories. Remember whatever you see in the camera viewfinder will be in the picture.

How to Position a Stillborn Baby in the Morgue

18. Positioning the baby in the morgue is very important. If the baby is not in good alignment with the head straight, pooling of blood occurs on the side of the face in which the head is turned. Proper positioning allows for subsequent viewings by the parents with little change in the baby's facial appearance and color. Use diaper rolls around the head and remainder of the body to promote good alignment.
Related: How to Photograph a Baby Not Alive

Our stillbirthday birth & bereavement doulas offer guidance in bathing and more.
[Used with permission, RTS Counselor Training Manual, 1993, p. 132]
Care providers can provide positive memories even when the stillborn's skin is compromised. Hopefully, these tips will provide some practical ideas. For more information, please call or write:
Bonnie K. Gensch, R.N. RTS Bereavement Coordinator Lutheran Hospital—La Crosse 1910 South Avenue La Crosse, WI 54601 Phone: 608-785-0530, ext. 3796
(This article was copied in its entirety from WiSSP)

HOW TO PHOTOGRAPH

Here are suggestions when photographing a baby not alive.

Photos as you enter the birth space:

- The parents' car
- The outside of birth place
- Nurses station or other signs to where the family are (maternity level or emergency room)
- The outside of birth room/room number
- Clock at intervals
- Parents after your introduction
- Any of their items/baby items
- Siblings or colorings from siblings (you can take a photo of their phone if they have any saved to that)
- Drinks, snacks, or other things that can serve to mark points of the labor, such as guests
- Parents – laughing, hugging, crying
- Crowning (hold in separate file for the mom)
- Early bonding
- As you leave, the clock or something outside to show the time change

To photograph the baby, here are some helpful tips:

- Begin taking pictures during pregnancy, the birth and as possible after birth. The physical form of the baby will change fast.
- Close-ups of the baby's hands and feet, and of the entire baby.
- You might include the parents' wedding rings, for size and to represent the special union which created the baby.
- You can include "props" like blankets, a flower or something meaningful to the family, and photograph the baby in different positions. A blanket can also be a beautiful way to cover parts of the baby with advanced physical changes while capturing a photo of hands or feet, for example.

Also Photograph:

- Every person impacted by the baby and present during whichever Season(s) you are capturing: Pregnancy, Birth, The Welcoming, The Farewell or The Healing Journey.
- Mom and/or Dad bonding with baby (reading, singing, touching, etc.).

During the Welcoming:

- Bonding.
- Actions including weighing & measuring.
- Items that touch the baby.
- Bathing and dressing.

Transitioning into the Farewell:

- Any keepsake making.
- Any staff present or parents on their phone.

Helpful tips about your camera, the photos, etc:

- Take time to read through and consider our pre-birth resource materials, including bonding in pregnancy, and creating the birth plan unique to this baby and this experience. These things can help create and capture meaningful events, feelings and experiences.
- Soften or shut off your flash. Using the light already in the room – window, computer screen glow, heat lamp, through the in-room bathroom, can be helpful.
- If you create both color and black and white copies, this lets the parents decide which they like.
- If you use editing software, keep copies of both versions so the family can choose. Trying to magnify the humanity of the baby while being realistic to what the family is actually seeing is important.
- Prepare the family to receive the photos – let them know you have them, and if possible, divide them between photos that can shape positive images of their experience, and the images that are more real, raw, or that you feel with your understanding of your time with them they may feel to be more private. These might be more graphic in nature. Hold a second copy of all photos in a safe place, for an amount of time you decide (1 year, 5 years, etc.), in the event that the originals become damaged.

If photographing the physical form of baby isn't possible:

- Perhaps in your birth experience, flushing was inevitable. The irretrievable birth of your baby's physical form into a bathroom basin can be for many mothers an extremely personal, painful and even traumatizing part of an already very painful experience. Please know that you are not alone. There are ways of speaking into this especially painful part of your journey with dignity and intention. Perhaps purposefully including water into your farewell can be especially redeeming, such as a love letter to your baby into a beautiful stream or ocean.
- Photographing aspects of the reality of baby in other ways can piece together into a very significant photo journal. The pregnancy test, the nursery, a baby outfit, a special place that you thought of or think of now when thinking of your baby, even if these things are purchased and photographed after the birth and death of your beloved baby, can bring validation and healing.
- We have more keepsake and farewell celebration ideas.
- We have more support for during the birth here.
- We have both short term and long term bereavement support resources for you here.

Additional Resources:
- ADEC_article
- Digital Photography
- Midwifery Today

My Notes

www.stillbirthday.com

POSTPARTUM HEMORRHAGE

If you are giving birth at home, it is important to be aware of the symptoms of a possible hemorrhage.

Hemorrhaging is a serious concern in at-home miscarriage, and may be enough reason for your care provider to discourage you from attempting to complete your miscarriage at home.

Generally, you will probably be cautioned that filling a regular-absorbancy maxi pad sooner than one hour, at any time, is cause of concern; immediately postpartum (that is, right after the baby is born), generally speaking you should not fill a regular-absorbancy maxi pad sooner than a half-hour in the first hour (so, you can go through 2 pads in the first hour postpartum), as it is common to experience some increased bleeding at the actual time of delivery.

An at-home aid in reducing blood loss may be found in a small amount of apple vinegar or 3 drops of cotton root bark applied directly to your tongue. This is something best discussed with your care provider while you are still laboring and before the birth.

If at any time you fill a maxi pad sooner than a half hour, experience dizziness, or a racing heart, you should consult a medical professional immediately.

If you are soaking through a maxi pad sooner than recommended by your medical provider, you need to seek medical attention (if you cannot reach your provider, please go to your nearest emergency room) immediately.
Medications that may be prescribed to help control the postpartum hemorrhage include:

- Misoprostol
- Methylergonovine

Misoprostol (a prostaglandin) causes your uterus to contract, so that your baby can be delivered. In addition, the prostaglandin works to block a hormone (progesterone) from completing its pregnancy function of supporting the uterine lining that the baby has been growing in. This will stop your body's efforts of sustaining the pregnancy.

"Cytotec" is one prescription name used, and misoprostol is said to have about an 80-90% effectiveness rate in delivering miscarried babies and completely expelling all of the placenta pieces. It is considered more effective than methylergonovine, but is not FDA approved for this use. For this reason, mothers may wish to request "Methergine" if it is considered a safer option by their provider.

Methylergonovine, commonly prescribed as "Methergine" is also a uterotonic; it causes your uterus to contract, which can shorten the duration of the delivery process, thus stopping the homorrhaging.

Your doctor will discuss with you the side effects and warning signs to look out for when taking these medications, and the amount of time it should take to complete the entire process.

Please visit our Levels of Augmentation article on herbal and natural alternatives to medications to help augment/speed up the time of the delivery of your miscarried baby.

Postpartum (all birth methods)

It is important to take care of yourself, both physically and emotionally, following a pregnancy loss. Regardless of the kind of pregnancy loss or the birth method you've used, it is important to replenish lost vitamins from blood loss and the birth. Here are a few helpful tips:

- Continue taking your prenatal vitamin.
- Ask your provider about floradix, hemoplex or chlorophyll, as these are said to have nourishing properties that can aid in replenishing lost iron and providing additional oxygenation to your blood.
- Stay hydrated.
- Salty broths can be satisfying and aid in lost iron.
- Vitamin C can help your body better absorb iron.
- Getting sunshine (even a one time trip to a tanning spa if it's winter) can help invigorate you.
- See the rest of our postpartum health tips.

www.stillbirthday.com

DONATING BREASTMILK

Breastmilk is a gift of life.

Getting Started

- know the options for donating, including legalities and fine print (outside link).
- understand that the desire to donate alone doesn't make it happen. Sometimes even if there is milk, it is not enough or the mother's body doesn't respond very well to pumping.
- discuss with your provider about the possibility of a discounted hospital pump rental.
- purchase or rent a pump.
- purchase comfortable nursing bras.
- purchase breastmilk storage bags.
- learn how to exclusively pump (including storage, hand expression, cleaning tools, and more).
- create a word file within a tag or business card template as explained below for easier labeling.
- keep receipts for your purchases as they may be needed in your donating arrangement.
- get support from your loved ones.
- If you want to pump and save or donate you milk, you will need support. It can be very hard to find the strength to keep going, but your support can help you go for as long as you would like to.

KEY TIPS:
• To keep an adequate supply, so you will be able to continue pumping for as long as you want to, pumping at least 8-12 times a day is necessary. Pumping every 2-3 hours will keep your supply up. Pump for up to 15 minutes on each side – do not pump endlessly even with small amounts of milk as this can fatigue the breast and actually dry the milk. You may hold near to you, baby lotion or another scent, or an item that belongs to baby, to help with "let-down". Household support by friends, and awareness for you to give validation to your spouse in other ways (such as listening, hand holding) can soften the sense of guilt which may accompany the spouse's desire for you to stop pumping.

• Find a bra that fits. Once you start to pump, get a fitting to see what size nursing bra will fit.
Most maternity stores will size women, but if you don't want to go into a store with pregnant women and newborns, you can look up how to size it yourself online or you can ask for help from your doula if you're is comfortable with it. Another great option is nursing tanks or tank tops. They will keep nursing pads in place, and make it easy to pump yet give support.

• Look into a hands-free pumping bra. Here is one brand. These are invaluable. When pumping exclusively, mothers are stuck to a pump for hours a day, and holding the pump in place gets exhausting, especially since pumping is pretty boring. A hands-free bra will let you pump, but also let you read or work while doing it. To go along with this, pumping makes you lean over into an unnatural position, and there are flanges (Pumpin' Pal) that go in the pump to lean the pump over while letting the mother relax.

• A good pump really helps ease the workload. If you would like to do this for longer than a month or two, you will need a pump that has the motor to sustain exclusive pumping. All hospital grade pumps will do this, though they are expensive. The Medela pumps aren't a closed pumping system so they aren't to be used for more than one person, but they are a good option. Hygeia pumps are the best pumps out there, and their professional grade pump are almost as powerful as hospital grade pumps for much cheaper. Ameda also has some amazing pumps to use.
• Drink a lot of water. Just the same as if you were nursing, you will need to drink water throughout the day to maintain her supply.

• Eat enough calories to stay healthy. One good rule of thumb is to eat 100 extra calories per 10 ounces pumped per day.

Pumping & Donating

• When storing milk, place the milk in whichever storage bag you have, and lie flat in your freezer until frozen. This takes up much less room in the freezer, so you can store more milk and it is much easier to transport. With some milk sharing arrangements, knowing on what day the milk was expressed is needed.

It might be simpler to create a word file with a tag or business card template that you can print multiple times, to include the following on each tag:

• Your name, day that your baby was born, at what week gestation he or she was born at, and a simple blank space or line for you to write on the date you expressed that batch of milk.

If donating, find someone to donate to once you have a supply or milk stored. There are many places to look for families to donate to. Eats on Feets and Human Milk 4 Human Babies are communities run through facebook, and you can just do a facebook search to find the chapter closest to you. These are both direct donation communities, so the donation is completely up to the families involved. Most should cover any expenses you had, such as storage bags or shipping.

• It may take a few days for the supply to rise, since the body wasn't prepared to make milk as early as it did. One way to increase supply is power pumping. This is more time consuming than pumping, but it works really well. When pumping, you pump for 5-10 minutes, then take a 5-10 minute break. Continue this for about an hour to an hour and a half, even if nothing else is coming out of the breast. The stimulation, even if nothing is coming out, will increase the supply. You can do this multiple times a day to increase it faster, but it is time consuming.
Mother's Milk is an herbal tea traditionally used to increase breastmilk production.

• Make sure that the flanges fit the breast. A lot of women don't have the average nipples and breasts required to fit the standard flanges (horns) on the breast pump. Lactation Innovation http://bit.ly/pZCCAS is a great resource to see if the flanges are the right size. If they are too big or small they can cause a lot of pain while pumping, clogged ducts, uneven emptying of the breast, and other issues. Correct flanges will help pumping be much less stressful.

• You will need support people, particularly a birth & bereavement doula, to be there, to check on you. It isn't easy to keep pumping, and there will be hard days when you may need someone to remind you why you started doing this. The benefits of breastmilk are endless, but after loss, it isn't that easy to remember why you started.

• If you donate your milk, the first time you drop off milk or milk is picked up can be hard. Your friends or a doula can ask if you will need them there, just for support. It is your baby's legacy and a wonderful thing for you to do, but it was also to be your own baby's nourishment.

If you ever have any questions, please do not hesitate to contact any of our birth & bereavement doulas, or our lactation professionals. Kayce Pearson pumped after her second trimester loss for two months, donated over 1000 ounces to three families, and encountered a lot of problems along the way, from clogged ducts to issues wanting to continue. Anytime you need help, you can send her a direct email. Kayce Pearson heartsandhandsservices@gmail.com Your loved ones will also need to provide support to you.

They can:
- bring or prepare meals for you.
- help with some of your basic household chores (laundry, for example).
- help run errands for you.
- not expect you to "host" or "entertain" them.
- visit our "friends/family" section for more helpful ideas.
- encourage you that you are making the right choice for your needs.
- remember that you are a new mom, which comes with a lot of needs, as well as a grieving mom, which also comes with a lot of needs.

Additional Information

This section is borrowed from "Expressing Breast Milk" written and revised by Edith Kernerman, IBCLC, and Jack Newman MD, FRCPC, IBCLC, and edited only to be appropriate for stillbirthday.

Obviously, if you can pump or express a lot of milk, you are producing a lot; however, if you cannot pump or express a lot, this does not mean your milk production is low or inadequate. Do not pump to find out how much you are producing. This is not a good way to judge milk supply.

The most effective pumps are high-powered, double, electric, and hospital-grade with adjustable pressure/suction and speed. There are many pumps on the market that are just not very good. Some hand pumps are adequate for occasional pumping.

Hand expression can be very effective and certainly is the least expensive. See below.
Improper use of a breast pump can lead to problems. Read all instructions thoroughly. Make sure you get a demonstration and instructions from the person who is renting or selling you the pump.

Pumping Method

Wash your hands.

Place your nipple in the center of the flange (when your baby is breastfeeding, it is best that your baby be latched on "off-centre" or "asymmetrically" with your nipple pointed toward the roof of baby's mouth (see the information sheet When Latching and the video clips.

Put the pump on the lowest setting that extracts milk, not the highest setting you can tolerate.

Pump for a maximum of 15 minutes each side. If breasts run "dry" before 15 minutes is up, pump until dry then add 2 minutes. Compression can be used when pumping as well and increases the amount you can pump. See the information sheet Breast Compression.

Remember, pumping should not hurt. If it hurts:
    Lower the suction setting
    Ensure the nipple is centered in the flange
    Pump for a shorter period of time

Cleaning the Pump

All pumping equipment should be sterilized before first usage, thereafter it only requires washing with hot, soapy, water or by dishwasher.

After each pumping: either place the pumping kit (not the tubes or motor) in the refrigerator until the next pumping, or if not pumping the same day, hot-water wash and hot-water rinse well, then air dry.

Remember to take apart all pieces of the pump for cleaning—including the smallest pieces, and to ensure that no milk has clumped in the flange shaft.

Hand Expression

Many mothers find that hand expression is an efficient way to pump when only occasional expression is required. In fact, when colostrum is present and the milk production is not abundant (as normal in the first few days), it is often easier to get milk with hand expression than with a pump and many mothers find this the easiest way to express mature milk as well.

- Wash your hands
- Place thumb and index finger on either side of the nipple, about 3 to 5 cm (1-2 inches) back from the nipple.
- Press gently inward toward the rib cage
- Roll fingers together in a slight downward motion
- Repeat all around the nipple if desired

Encouraging the milk ejection reflex (MER) or "let down" reflex

The milk ejection reflex or "let down" reflex is the sudden rushing down of the milk. Milk will flow quickly even if you are not pumping at the time. Some mothers may feel thirsty, sweaty, sleepy, or dizzy during a milk ejection reflex. However, many mothers do not feel this milk ejection response ever in their whole lactating experience. You do not need to feel or be aware of the milk ejection reflex in order for there to be milk. Some women only become aware of it after the first few weeks while others feel it only at the beginning and no longer do after the first few weeks. This has absolutely no bearing on milk supply.

You can encourage the milk ejection reflex by thinking about having your baby in your arms or at your breast or having a picture of your baby to look at or keeping a piece of his clothing next to you.

You may feel the milk ejection reflex or notice your breasts leaking or you may not. You are likely to pump more milk faster if you pump both breasts at the same time. Breast compressions, while pumping, can be very effective at increasing the amount expressed, it may be a bit awkward at first, but it can be done (mothers have fixed the cups so that they sit inside the bra and then use compressions) or the partner can do it.

SHARING THE LEGACY OF MILK

Understand the pain medication options your providers might offer you and how these might interfere with your lactation options.

Undergo a screening like at a Milk Bank.*
Having a doula or friend with you, especially for your first drop-off is important, as well as having something tangible you might hold during the exchange.

About Milk Donation – Screening*
All donors to a HMBANA Milk Bank undergo a screening process that begins with a short telephone interview.

Donor mothers must be:

- in good health
- not regularly on most medications or herbal supplements (with the exception of prenatal vitamins, human insulin, thyroid replacement hormones, nasal sprays, asthma inhalers, topical treatments, eye drops, progestin-only or low dose estrogen birth control products; for other exceptions, please contact a milk bank for more information).
- willing to undergo blood testing (at the milk bank's expense)
- willing to donate at least 100 ounces of milk (some banks have a higher minimum)

You would not be a suitable donor if you:

- use illegal drugs
- smoke or use tobacco products
- have received a blood transfusion or blood products (except Rhogam) in the last 4 months
- have received an organ or tissue transplant in the last 12 months
- regularly have more than 2 ounces of alcohol per day
- have a positive blood test result for HIV, HTLV, hepatitis B or C, or syphilis
- or your sexual partner is at risk for HIV
- have been in the United Kingdom for more than 3 months (1980-96)
- have been in Europe for more than 5 years (1980-present)

Donated milk is heat processed (pasteurized) to remove potentially harmful bacteria and viruses.

Join the SBD Milk Sharing Map
If you are sharing your baby's legacy of milk, if you are in need of breastmilk, or if you are a lactation support resource, you can list your information on our Milk Sharing Map.
SOURCE OF DOCUMENT:http://www.stillbirthday.com/2011/10/20/post-loss-lactation-2/

DRYING BREASTMILK

In between the two options of donating or drying breastmilk, you may have even just a few droplets of breastmilk that you might save onto a cloth nursing pad, or create into a jewelry item, or, you may still be nursing an older toddler and can cherish the shared gift.

The options for support and for validating your experience are many.

This following information comes as it's foundation from Kayce Pearson, SBD

• Do not bind off the breasts. This can cause clogged ducts and can lead to infection and mastitis. This includes tight bras like sports bras or tight tank tops.

• One of the best natural remedies is cabbage leaves in the bra. Just take regular cabbage leaves, either the entire leaf or cut since it needs to fit over most of the breast, and fit it in the bra. Make sure that if the entire leaf doesn't cover, put some on both sides of the breast. This will evenly decrease the milk supply without causing clogged ducts or any other issues. If this is done around the clock, most see a huge decrease within a couple days. Change out the leaves twice a day for the best effect. [preparing the leaves by cutting off the biggest veiny sections, and then placing them in freezer bags in the freezer, and changing them out once they become warm and soggy, can provide relief from the physical pain of engorgement as well as helping to dry the milk quickly.]

Ice can be your best friend. When decreasing supply, engorgement can happen. Using ice doesn't stimulate supply, and it helps take the edge off any pain they can be experiencing. Earth Mama Angel Baby makes Booby Tubes, which are great for this. They can be frozen or heated, and curl around the breast so all the sore parts are covered.

Earth Mama Angel Baby also makes No More Milk tea. Peppermint and sage also can help lower breastmilk supply. Try not to stimulate the breasts at all. Any stimulation, such as rubbing in the shower, can signal the breasts to make more milk. However, if the breast is really engorged, hand expressing until comfortable can really help, as long as it isn't done every few hours.

09.
LOVED ONES:
FAMILY & FRIENDS
AND PROVIDERS

FAMILY & FRIENDS

It can be terribly uncomfortable, wanting to offer support to parents of a lost child, but not knowing the best way to do it. Sometimes very well meaning and loving expressions can actually be received as insulting and damaging. To prevent this, here is a helpful list of ideas for you to consider:

Helpful Things You Might Know:

You can be a much needed support prior to, during (yes, that's right, during), or after birth in any trimester. Research proves that the level of grief a parent experiences is not conditional upon the age of the child. Meaning, younger children are "worth" just as much grief as older children.

Mothers who experience pregnancy & infant loss are at risk of developing postpartum major depression. The risk of this depression is highest within the first six months after birth. The mothers who are at greatest risk of becoming depressed are those who fail to show any signs of grief during the first two weeks after the birth (source).

Experiencing pregnancy & infant loss in a way that demonstrates the reality of your baby's life, and death, is actually important to your postpartum health.

Men and women experience grief differently. Supportive efforts might be helpful for one parent more than the other. We have support for dads here, too.

Grief can be ongoing, can seem unpredictable, and can take time. Parents remember their children for the rest of their lives.

You and your bereaved loved one may benefit greatly from you learning about their type of loss and the other information we share here at stillbirthday, including support for getting pregnant again, support for surviving siblings, facing a struggle with fertility, and more.

The parents at highest risk of complications in their emotional healing are those that show no signs of grief in the first two weeks following the death of their child.

The actual loss is only the beginning of a journey of grief. The four most difficult times following a pregnancy loss are often: the return of the first menstrual cycle, the month in which the gender of the baby would have been discovered, the due date for the full term delivery, and the timeframe of the first anniversary of the loss (first stillbirthday). Holidays within the first year can also be painful, particularly Mother's Day/Father's Day (and/or Bereaved Mothers/Bereaved Fathers days), Thanksgiving and Christmas. Mothers too can face climactic milestones in subsequent pregnancy and birth. It is extremely positive to remember these times and reach out to your loved ones during at least one of these, offering to share an afternoon together or just to let them know that you care.

Grief can include a full range of feelings, at any time, including happiness and relief. Grief isn't bound by blue or grey but can be every color of the rainbow.

You may be grieving, too, and may benefit from utilizing long term support services.

If the couple has other children, there is information and support for older siblings at stillbirthday in our grief support resources.

Honoring the privacy of the parents is important, but so is being able to communicate your own grief. For that reason, we have a section here where you can share your story (and read other stories), and it will be published in the category of "friends & family". Your story can bless others in a similar situation, without overstepping the privacy that the parents may have requested. We ask that you do not use their real names in your story.

Grandparents grieve too. AGAST is one organization for grandparent grief.

Stillbirthday has helpful resources for grandparents, fathers, surviving and subsequent children:Emotional/Spiritual Support.

Crisis Lines, Books, Websites (some by country) can be helpful for you to know for the parents.

Helpful Things You Might Bring:

Bring A Love Basket, for the earliest and darkest days.

These are suggested items, and may be brought by more than one loved one:

- buy a special gown (particularly from Bg&Co) for the mother to give birth in
- gather information for the mother on prior to birth, during birth, and after birth
- understand about postpartum items and support she may need, including maxi pads for lochia, and items to support her decision regarding breastmilk (including donation)
- buy a small or medium sized package of heavy maxi pads for the mom (birth in any trimester can mean a lot of bleeding)
- bring a meal (or two) that is easy to prepare (more information on this below)
- bring healthful, easy to munch snacks that can aid in healthy grieving
- buy a teddy bear or other gift, particularly prior to or during the birth, so that the mother won't have to leave the place of her child's birth empty-handed – see our craft idea with teddy bears below
- give the mother a gift card (not a huge amount, $20 would be great) to her favorite shop or a clothing store
- buy the mom a comfortably-fitting blouse that is non-maternity (especially if she was further along in pregnancy)
- include a card that shares your sorrow and includes the baby's name, as well as lists any other tangible ways you are available to help, including babysitting surviving children, mowing, shoveling snow, folding a load of laundry or any other simple tasks.

Meal Tips:

- Make enough for leftovers.
- Consider the older children and their tastes. Including a McDonald's gift card can be helpful.
- Write reheating instructions if necessary.
- Bring a gallon of milk, a loaf of fresh bread and a fruit basket so that basic groceries aren't needed.
- Do not send meals in a dish you need returned.
- Call before you go.
- Mailing a card with a restaurant gift card is a nice alternative as well.
- These ideas and a beautiful story are shared at Cooker & a Looker

Other Helpful Things You Might Do:

- Has your friend invited you to support her during the actual birth?
- Learn some foundational tips on serving as a doula where birth & bereavement meet.
- hire an SBD doula or an SBD chaplain
- host a Celebrating Pregnancy blessingway /Stillbirthday Sacred Circle (strongly recommended, even if this is done after the birth of the baby)
- consider our book list for loved ones in how to support through grief
- consider our many keepsakes and jewelry items
- buy a special gift acknowledging her loss (the comfort company has many ideas)
- participate in any farewell celebration the family might be participating in
- clean, tidy the home, do a load of laundry, bring in their mail, mow their lawn
- attend any foll0w-up doctor's visits with the mom
- talk about the baby by name
- send a card to the family at the first birthday or another holiday. Lost for Words is one card line specific to pregnancy and infant loss, or a Birth Verse card
- sign up for another grieving mother to send her hand written letters through the Joy Comes in the Morning project
- buy a helpful book for the parents (see our list of books)
- consider the mom's interpretation of your gestures
- visit the Farewell Celebrations page, as there are gift ideas there as well

Honor the Dad & Other Children:

Our Momentos section has special keepsakes for Stillbirthday Fathers and Children.
Sharing our Fathers & Children resources could be very helpful.
Supporting the couple so that he is emotionally available to explore the birth and death of his child from his own perspective, rather than serving entirely in a protective role for his wife, is helpful.

Craft Idea:

Find out from the mother how much her baby weighs.
Measure out that weight in rice. If you don't have an ounce scale at home, bring your rice to the grocery store. Check in with a cashier or another employee first to be sure there isn't any confusion about theft or anything like that.
Measure out the weight in rice, using a small plastic baggie to hold the rice.
Purchase a teddy bear. A Build-A-Bear would work very well.
Carefully cut the back seam of the bear, remove a small amount of the stuffing, and place the baggie of rice into the bear. Sew up the seam.
Now the mom has a bear that weighs as much as her baby.
Incorporating a small pouch and zippered back as an alternative, to hold small keepsakes like the baby's hospital bracelet or a love letter to the baby, is also a loving idea.

Helpful Things You Might Say:

- *I want to know* – in word or action, this could be the most important sentiment to convey. This individual mother, father or surviving sibling knows the most of their own experience, and coming alongside them in a way that is slow, that is curious, that is trusting, allows them to explore what the situation means to them, and allows them to express what the situation means to them. The most important thing you might say is nothing at all, but opening up a safe place to listen. You will not at all know how to come alongside this mother and this family if you do not take the time to know who this mother and family are – how do they interpret their experiences, what are their spiritual beliefs, what are their needs.
- In our doula training, we teach this fundamental "series" of support: slow down, validate, provide options and supplement resources. To support well, you don't have to support alone. Be prepared to wrap the mother in support options and know of a few resources that match her needs.
- I'm sorry
- Your feelings are OK. (This might be followed with:) If your feelings get scary or dangerous, a counselor or pastor can help you navigate them. I can help you find one.
- I don't know if she asks why it happened. Don't guess or assume.
- I miss (name of baby) too or I wanted to know (name of baby) too. This should not be said in a way that suggests grief comparison or makes the parent feel guilty for "feeling too much", but should be said in a loving way of sharing the grief together.

If you have experienced a pregnancy & infant loss yourself, prior to fairly recent years:

- In honor both of your own experience, and/or the recent loss that was experienced by your loved one, you may wish to join our mentorship program.
- Your perception of care for pregnancy & infant loss may likely be very different than the care that is given today. You may recall any of the following in your own experience: not seeing your baby, not holding your baby, not naming your baby, not knowing where your baby was buried, not knowing if your baby was given his or her own grave. You may not have ever talked about your experience, although the pain and reality of the death of your baby is real. Please consider sharing your story with us. Your story will also be categorized in the "prior to 1990's" section if applicable.
- MISS Foundation offers grief support for grandparents ("AGAST").
- You may become jealous or confused at the care and attention that is given to mothers and families who experience loss today. There are positive, healthy ways to work through these feelings without projecting any negative feelings onto the couple as they endure their grief now. Please visit the long term support resources for ideas.
- You can contact your local Vital Statistics office for information on your stillbirth experience so that you may have some deeper healing and closure to your own experience.

If you are pregnant, while a loved one is experiencing bereavement:

- Consider sharing the news with your friend privately, and before you share the news with others. This allows her to process the information privately, and gives her control.
- Acknowledge the very real grief that your loved one is enduring, and recognize that she may have many mixed feelings about your pregnancy. She may likely be genuinely happy for you, but this joy will likely be mixed with jealousy and hurt, and at different times in your pregnancy these feelings may be magnified. Validate to your loved one what you expect from her feelings, and let her know that she can discuss these things, either with you or with other support such as a counselor or pastor. Refer her to the long term support resources section for more information.
- When planning your baby shower, discuss her invitation with her privately, preferably before the other invitations go out. Let your loved one know that she is invited and her presence will be meaningful to you, but that you acknowledge that it may be upsetting for her, and that you'd like to give her room to make her own choice regarding attending. She may like to give a gift separately instead of attending.
- If you are a long distance from the family:
- In addition to many of the above suggestions, Caring from a Distance has ideas you may be able to incorporate into your support.

Things That Would Not Be Helpful To Do Or Say

Things that would not be helpful to do:

- remove, pack up, or destroy items from the baby room without both parents' permission
- petition the mother in any way to celebrate anybody else's pregnancy or baby, until the mother initiates interest herself, or at least several weeks have passed

Things that would not be helpful to say:

- One in Two Won't offers a little video, so that you can hear the things not to say.
- Giving any explanation whatsoever (medical or speculation) is generally not a good idea.
- Pointing out that the mother has more time to have children. Right now, she is grieving this child (and, conception may have taken longer than you know).
- Pointing out that the mother has more children – either older siblings or multiples of the baby who didn't survive (unless her grief is becoming destructive, and more professional assistance is suggested to help).
- Promoting the idea that a twinless twin is a singleton, for example, or that two surviving babies from a set of triplets are instead twins (seeming or attempting to ignore the reality of all of the multiples in the pregnancy).
- Suggesting in any way that this is a positive or a good outcome.
- Pressuring the mother or the father to grieve differently than they are. Please see our resources on different grieving styles.
- Initiating or engaging in controversial discussions with either parent on topics such as elective abortion or some kinds of fetal research. This can serve to invalidate the grief the parent is experiencing – even regardless of their general or prior position on such topics. It may be wise to pick a different topic, or pick a different person to discuss it with.
- Attempting to participate in decisions such as telling the couple they should start trying to conceive immediately, or offering discouragement at the news of a subsequent pregnancy.
- Suggesting in any way that this outcome is the fault of the mother (or father), unless you are gently and compassionately offering support resources for an obviously risky situation that you know for certain occured during the pregnancy (ie drug abuse, domestic violence). Remember, offering general speculation is not a good idea.
- Anything with just, said or implied, is hurtful. "You can just have more children, you should just get over it…"
- Telling the parents where you believe their baby's soul or spirit to be can be received offensively regardless of their faith. Allow the parent the right to explore answers of life after death without belittling them or minimizing the reality of the death of their baby. In addition, attention to where the baby is, is only part of the care that a mother needs. It is extremely important to remember that she is here – she is without her child – and she is hurting.

PROVIDER CARE

When you are a provider, and you are the mother enduring loss:

When you endure loss personally, the impact of your experience can touch every way you are connected to birth, both personally and professionally. One such way is a subsequent loss of passion for birth work. This loss of passion for birth work, can include any number of things. Here's just 5 to consider:

- Jealousy of other mothers.

- Suppressing your story out of fear of scaring mothers.

- Suppressing your story out of fear of being invalidated, scorned, or reprimanded for "fear mongering", "not having enough faith in birth" or "not getting over your loss."

- Suppressing your story out of fear that it contradicts your stance on ____, which can be absolutely any single thing related in any way whatsoever to pregnancy, birth or motherhood, including but not limited to, for examples: pro-life v. pro-choice, medicalized birth assistance (how does needing a D&C impact your professional stance on hands-off birth, for example.

- Unsubstantiated but heightened fear or paranoia in labors (a kind of "fear of jinxing").

Your journey in healing requires that you go slow, to spend time in exploring how you define your experience personally, without any boundaries set by others or even by yourself professionally. Only then can you begin to discover how your experience might integrate into your professional role in the positive, enriching and holistic ways in which it absolutely has the potential to. Spend some time here at stillbirthday looking at the resources and support specifically through the lens of the mother you are. When you are ready, you are invited to share your story, either through the main sharing page or here, at the end of this page (just scroll down). There are no expectations here, no requirements that you know, feel, say or do anything. You are free to explore your own experience authentically. You are worthy, and, you aren't alone.

"I had been a doula for 10 years, when I gave birth to my baby in the first trimester...
"...And even at that, I was still so alone, so ill prepared..."

When you are the provider, supporting a client enduring loss:

Stillbirthday aims to provide compassion and support to all providers who are impacted by patient or client loss, including:

- doulas
- hospice workers
- leaders of pregnancy loss organizations
- mentors or counselors or chaplains
- ultrasound technicians
- paramedic professionals
- nurses
- midwives
- doctors
- if you are a birth educator (author, teacher, social media user, or in any other capacity), stillbirthday interviewed several professionals to bring you helpful information for broaching the subject of pregnancy loss

In Provider Care, the provider comes first – and that's you!

We do this in three parts: get support, be support, and share.

1. Get Support

a.) Provider Care {Mentoring} Program

- **Mentoring resources for the professional:**
- Stillbirthday provides a uniquely designed significant resource for all birth & bereavement professionals in our Provider Care program.

b.) Events

- Check our events page for things you can get involved in or encourage others to.
- Our Workshop for Birth Professionals
- You can schedule an event with any of our Executive Team, including Heidi Faith, to speak.

c.) Other Online Materials

Please also utilize this list of articles that pertain to things such as compassion fatigue or other information regarding how to care for yourself as the provider:

- How to Doula in Bereavement gives you practical tools to support the family, and yourself
- Take our brief, confidential survey to share how you or your team generally responds to client/patient fetal demise.
- Check update educational information from our Official Affiliates
- Nurse.com : Good Grief (external link)
- Workingnurse.com : How to Grieve Well (external link)
- Nurses Mentoring developed by CHOP (external link)
- Secondary Traumatic Stress (STS) and Compassion Fatigue
- Midwives can join the ACNM eMidwife Discussion Groups
- Self-Compassion article
- Obstetricians experience guilt and stress
- Medical providers grieve after making mistakes
- Jealousy in Birth Workers (we discuss additional factors in our training as well)

Give yourself time to grieve. Whether your professional experience is one loss in your entire career, or, one loss a week, you need time to process what happened. Even if the death of a baby is a common occurance in your work, the death of a baby is not normal. Process the events so that you don't reflect feelings of fear of death toward patients or clients who will not experience loss.

As the provider or professional involved, you may face feelings of guilt, whether or not you provided your care to the best of your skill level and ability or not. Please, be gentle on yourself. Blame can be a natural reaction from the family. Their feelings are part of their process and they will need to work through them. You also need to work through your own feelings, of guilt, or blame. Remember that feelings of guilt or blame are secondary to the reality that a baby died. A baby died, and grief is involved - the family's, and yours. Reading our interview with a midwife on this subject might be helpful for you.

Homebirth Loss Awareness Day

You will likely still reflect and assimilate the situation, whether there are feelings of guilt or not. Be sure to do this in a healthy, positive way, looking to affirm honestly the ways in which you are a good provider – and, a growing provider.

Seek additional support for yourself, through our many resources here at stillbirthday, including our long term support, which is listed according to location as well as crisis hotlines, websites and books. Remember that you can best care for the family when you are cared for yourself.

Take the Psychology Today Burnout Exam.

2. Be Support.

a.) Get Professionally Trained

- SBD Birth & Bereavement Training

b.) Other Online Materials

You of course need to provide support for the mother and the family. Here are a few tips:

- "I Want To Know"

- Make this your mantra, in word and action.

- Visit our birth plan section for ways to support the family immediately from the time of birth, helping the mother navigate her many postpartum experiences and choices, and visit our Family/Friends section for many ways that you can provide support.

Prior to loss

Prepare your environment for birth in any trimester.

A laboring room specifically for miscarriage in the Emergency Room as well as a room especially for loss on L&D is an appropriate and realistic investment into the longterm health of your community.

The laboring room should have resources present for the immediate experience, including items that may help identify and preserve the physical form of the baby.

The laboring room should not have an auto-flush toilet.

The laboring room should also have resources present for long term and follow up postpartum as well as grief support.

Families should be privy to their personal options regarding birth in any trimester, with any level of medical support and in any outcome. This includes information regarding options they do have regarding D&C or other medically assisted birth.

There should not be gaps or overlaps in care. These cause chasms that families fall into. Have a direct relationship with some of your local community resources, including funeral home staff, SBD doulas and social workers.

During birth and/or death

Go slow. Validate. Provide Options. Supplement Resources.

Language is Important.

As you issue a death notification, go slow. Learn how to give the death notification to this particular family. Be aware: determine if your patient, and all present with her, is in a safe position and situation to receive the death notification. Be curious: get to eye level with the mother, rather than looming over her. Be specific: I cannot find a heartbeat, Sue. Be clear: give facial expression and body presence that show nearness, compassion, and a curiosity to listen to her response. Be ready: be ready to repeat the news. Be ready to give time.

Words shared by mothers who found them hurtful, include: just a period, product of conception, debris, spontaneous abortion, terminating, removal, dispose of, try again, mood disorder.

Finding a cause, which can include blame, is only part of what the family is enduring. Learn how to accept words without internalizing the message.

Mirror the reactions the family is displaying to you regarding their experience.

After loss

Take our brief, confidential survey to share how you or your team generally responds to client/patient fetal demise.

Telling the mother "I'm sorry for your loss" is not a legally binding statement and does not suggest liability. Do not be afraid to say "I'm sorry for your loss."

Hug the mother, and cry with her. Let the family mourn. Mourning is the outward demonstration of the internalized feeling of grief.

If giving the mother time to process her experience and her choices is at all a possibility, please do so. If you are sharing the news of an impending pregnancy loss or a difficult diagnosis, don't pressure the mother while you explain what her options may be.

Help coordinate in the immediate events – for example, if this was a homebirth, please visit our home stillbirth page

Help coordinate the longterm events – for example, if the baby has a fatal diagnosis

Ask to attend the funeral or other Farewell Celebration

Help the mother prepare for what to expect during the birth. Stillbirthday has many resources to help with this, particularly in our birth plan section, which links to things like giving the baby a bath and what to expect from the appearance of the baby's skin.

Help the mother and family with special momentos and keepsakes. If the mother refuses to see her baby or take photos, ask if you can take photos in a nearby room, and include any willing family members. Offer other momentos such as a lock of the baby's hair. If the family does not want these keepsakes, ask if you can store them for the family as they may wish for them at a later time.

Don't tell the mother, "You should have…. (called me sooner)"

Don't tell the mother, "Your baby…(did this to himself)"

Don't tell the mother, "I'm sorry you think I did something to cause this." This is minimizing, and focuses on what you may believe to be projection, rather than the reality that her baby has died. Say instead, "I'm sorry that your baby has died. I am here, and I will help you navigate testing and find out what happened."

If you are or believe you may be at fault somehow, don't dwell on that. Assure the mother that medical testing will answer those questions. Again, "I don't know why this happened, but I am here with/for you."

Help the mother seek medical answers for her loss if she wishes, including additional testing and perinatologist or other professional referrals

Continue with postpartum care, including physical and emotional care. Our birth plans section provides information on things like breastmilk decisions, Cesarean birth recovery, as well as how to navigate the sometimes conflicting aspects of the Farewell Celebrations and the physical postpartum healing of the mother (for example, how to plan a funeral in the event of a Cesarean birth, so that the mother can attend).

View our "Outside Insight" section of articles for more ideas on how to support well.

Remember, all the resources above are also for your benefit. How to Doula in Bereavement gives you practical tools to support the family, and yourself.

Every level professional can benefit greatly from taking stillbirthday's birth & bereavement training program.

3. Share

Take our brief, confidential survey to share how you or your team generally responds to client/patient fetal demise.

You also have the opportunity to submit stories and share your experiences with others. You can read these stories here, at the "Provider Care" category of stories. This can be a very healing way to let mothers know that providers also grieve the losses of those they support, and can give other professionals important insight into helpful ways to support during loss, and helpful ways to process and heal through the experiences. You can also share of your support with "rainbow/subsequent" pregnancies.

A few very important things to know when you submit a story to be published at stillbirthday:

HIPAA is a priority. See Permitted Uses numbers 3 and 4, along with "De-Identified Health Information". You should consider having the written consent of the mother prior to sharing your story, although it is not a requirement. These stories can be seen by mothers.

When you submit a story, your name is omitted. It will read that it was contributed anonymously.

Any and all names of people involved are omitted and/or altered.

Any reference to time that can be an identifying factor ("Three months ago...") will be omitted.

Any reference to medical or other public facilities, or other identifying factors will be omitted.

Additional information may be also be altered or omitted.

If a mother believes she has identified herself in any story, and objects to its publication, it will be removed immediately. You can view our additional submission information.

10.
FAREWELL CELEBRATIONS

www.stillbirthday.com

FAREWELL CELEBRATIONS

There are ways to honor your little one, regardless of just how little he or she is.
These ideas are specific to recognizing the life and death of your baby – at any time, including funeral planning and keepsake items to purchase from different organizations. There are also many personalized birth plan options to help you celebrate the life of your baby during the labor and delivery.

Celebrating
A very young, unrecognizable baby:
A baby not buried:
A baby from a long time ago:

- Celebrating Pregnancy Blessingway – Stillbirthday Sacred Circles
- SBD Chaplains have many special, unique alternative cremation and burial options. These can be very difficult decisions but it can be very important to know that you have options you may not otherwise know about. SBD Chaplains use tools and resources including small cast iron pots, fruit dehydrators and many more ideas that are available simply for you to consider.
- placenta burial
- unofficial burial (including baby clothing and casket information).
- farewell words and music (can be included in the unofficial burial)
- Using a very small piece of paper or colored tissue paper, you can draw a picture or write a note and flush that during the time of your bleeding. Or, you can release flower petals or a love letter to your baby into a stream. Many stillbirthday mothers value incorporating water into their farewell when flushing was inevitable.
- Some funeral homes offer a memorial wall or garden for names of babies who are not buried there.
- Confirm with your local crisis pregnancy center that they can and should offer ultrasounds for every mother enduring an impending miscarriage, as this may be the only photo she will have of her baby, and consider donating to their organization if they do offer such a valuable service to bereaved families.
- Donate to your SBD doula or to our SBD doula sponsorship program to equip more doulas to serve families.
- Donate to an organization or business that offers discounted or free pregnancy & infant loss resources (such as Mason's Cause or AngelNames.org).
- Raise funds for your local perinatal or pediatric hospice/palliative care.
- Volunteer to help minister to and encourage other mothers: here are important tips to consider when resolving to get involved.
- Place a birth and/or death announcement in your local newspaper so that you can keep that for your own keepsake.
- Create a birth or a death announcement (or both) in a postcard or other format. We offer an online version at stillbirthday.
- Birth & Bereavement Activism, Art & Expression.
- Blog about your story or in other ways reach out and share your experience.
- Share your experience with us here at this site (we'd be honored and blessed).
- Spread the word offers a "Blog Button" and other ways to help others including our Debris Day.
- Order a stillbirthday cake.
- Special remembrance jewelry (See our list! There's a lot!)
- Special momentos (See our list! There's a lot!)

- Release a balloon, perhaps with a small letter or prayer attached.
- Please see our birth plans for a full section of birth planning, birth, and immediate postpartum support, including, for example, items from Earth Mama Angel Baby.
- Purchasing an unofficial Certificate of Birth as a momento. Portraits by Dana offers one as well. (Stillbirthday has a free Certificate of Birth basic template).
- Incorporating water into your farewell, particularly when flushing is inevitable:
- Seashore of Remembrance
- Sacred Water Offering

Celebrating

An identifiable baby:
An older baby:

- Any of the above ideas for a smaller baby.
- See your state listing of professionals/volunteers for photographers in your area.
- Consider breastmilk donation (and get help from the hospital staff with nursing).
- Investigate as soon as possible if your state offers an official certificate of stillbirth.
- Visitation at hospital, home, or funeral.
- Farewell words and music (can be included in the funeral).
- Official, cemetary burial options (including hospital cremation, funeral home cremation, funeral, clothing, and casket information).
- If you have baby items or the nursery already set up, do not pack anything away until both parents agree to this decision. If at that time you decide that you'd like to share your baby's items with others, Missing Solace has a Christmas present donation program. You can also participate in our Love Cupboard program.
- Special momentos for older babies (see our list! There's a lot!)

Honoring Stillbirthday Fathers

Dads can honor the real life and the real death of their babies in special and unique ways, including any of the above ideas. For more suggestions, visit our:

☐ family and friends/ gift ideas for dads
☐ support resources for dads

Things that may not be very helpful

Believing or acting as though the burial location is a nursery or that the baby is somehow living there.
Volunteering for long-term projects in your baby's name, because if you cannot follow through you may be left with tremendous guilt.
Naming a pet or another child the same name as your lost child, unless both parents fully agree to this.

If you've experienced loss in the past

You may know someone who's lost a baby many years ago, and never thought there were options for their family to honor their little one. No time or distance can deter a mother from celebrating the life, and death, of her child. If you are that mother, you can still honor your child. You can choose from different items on this page, too, in particular, the ones for celebrating a very young baby.

Cultural Farewell Traditions & Customs & Burial Items

- Our SBD Chaplains can officiate the farewell celebration of your choosing, as well as guiding you in caring for your baby's physical form and preparing for natural burial. All of our SBD Chaplains are also trained SBD Doulas, which means that they can also support you prior to and during your birth, as well as support your postpartum needs. You can visit the "During Birth" resources for a listing of your local SBD Doulas and SBD Chaplains.
- Burial Shrouds
- Hindu
- Muslim
- Native American
- Burial Jewelry
- Baha'i
- Matching Mother/Child Jewelry (one buried with baby, one kept and worn by mother)
- Birth Verse
- B'earth Angel

Cultural and religious information pertaining to bereavement (including cultural keepsakes) can be found in our Long Term Healing Perspectives section.

11.

THE LONGTERM HEALING JOURNEY

THE HEALING JOURNEY

For Mothers~

The earliest moments of encountering the realization that your baby is not alive can be the most catastrophically overwhelming and quite literally the most traumatizing moments of your life.

You are still a mother. You are still worthy of giving birth to your beloved baby, and your precious one will be born. If I can just encourage you with that, it would be that you are a beautiful mother, and that you matter.

Please, even in this impossible time, go slow.
Ask questions. Ask for support.

The experience of pregnancy and infant loss doesn't end when your baby is born. You will be for the rest of your life a mother. And for the rest of your life, you are worthy of healing.

When you are ready, make yourself a warm cup of cocoa or fresh lemonade, snuggle in your pajamas and pull up your computer. Type in www.stillbirthday.com.

The purple bar across the top of the screen guides you in chronological order, from support prior to birth – including explanations of medical terms, and what to expect from the birth method your medical provider deems safest for you.

The "during support" resources will lead you into hundreds of pages, similar to those in this book. Birth plan preparations including questions to ask your care team, information about alternatives and how to connect with a local doula, all are there.

Mothers who have embarked on this journey before you have allowed stillbirthday to hold their babies' photos, and their birth stories. From every week gestation to particular special and unique aspects of their stories, mothers, fathers, siblings and loved ones from all over the world have shared their stories at stillbirthday that you might know you are not alone.

There are events, news articles, research and interpretive resources for spiritual support and psychological understanding of bereavement, contributed poems, and more, all for you.

I am so very sorry for your loss and for what you may be enduring.

May you know simply that you are loved.

MY LONGTERM HEALING JOURNEY

Ways I have already grown:
_____
_____

Areas I've forgiven others:
_____
_____

Areas I've forgiven myself:
_____
_____

New support I've discovered:
_____
_____

Unexpected challenges I have met:
_____
_____

Unexpected support I have encountered:
_____
_____

Goals I have:
_____
_____

MORE OF MY THOUGHTS
_____
_____
_____
_____
_____
_____
_____
_____
_____

FOR FURTHER EXPLORATION
Words from Heidi's Heart

Subsequently

On the hot summer night of June 7, several years ago, a woman began to labor her child, her daughter. The father of the child lay asleep in the bedroom, after leaving stern instruction not to be awakened unless the birth of the child was imminent.

She labored, alone, quietly, until she was sure it was time to wake him.

In the dark morning of June 8, she mounted his motorcycle, this laboring mother, and held the back of his leather jacket as he rode her to the hospital entrance. Prior to "The Bradley Method" of childbirth, which includes the father in the laboring process, was the "Jack Daniels Method"; the man rode on to the nearest bar to celebrate the arrival of his daughter. The woman entered the hospital, alone.

This same woman labored two years earlier, and gave birth to a stillborn little girl.

What was this labor like for her? Was she scared? Terrified of what might happen? Did her body's successive pulls and squeezes, painful contractions, remind her of when she had experienced this last? Did she pray? Did she hope? Did she cry? Did she long for someone to wipe her forehead with a cool, damp cloth and tell her that her feelings are OK, that everything is going to be OK? Did she wonder if this little girl she was about to meet would be breathing, would look at her, see her, respond to her touch, or if this little girl, like her last, would die during birth?

I don't know.

She never told me. Pieces of my childhood are jotted down in notes – notes in different handwriting from the different people who made executive decisions on my behalf. I don't know how my mother felt about my birth, because her feelings aren't jotted down in my government issed file. It is probable that nobody bothered to ask her.

A short time after my birth, my mother went to prison and my father fled the state. I was raised in foster care, group homes, and institutions for the majority of my childhood.

What if someone had intervened? What if someone had wiped her forehead with a cool cloth, and told her it was OK to feel what she was feeling? What if, before this pregnancy, someone offered her mentorship after my older sister had died?

Would she and my father have begun to seek a healthy, legal lifestyle? Would she have escaped his abuses and began a life of healing?

Mothers of miscarried and stillborn babies need immediate support. We need support at the exact time of the news that the baby is not going to live. We need support through the remainder of the pregnancy, and through the process of childbirth. We need postpartum support. These things are, in large part, what our bereavement doula program is all about. And, we need support long after these things are over.

Our doula and mentorship programs may not be enough to stop a predisposition for addictions and abuses, but it could be enough to reveal these predispositions and it could be enough to recognize the hunger for healing. It could change lives.

Furthermore, a parent's life is forever changed after the birth of a stillborn baby and many, many mothers who've given birth to miscarried babies recognize this same irreparable break.

We will never be the same.

It is a new beginning. A new birth. A new life. A subsequent life.

In the same way newborns need to be cradled, held close, and touched tenderly, so too are bereaved mothers. Sometimes, we can walk. Sometimes we crawl, and still other times we just need to be carried. But we always want our loved ones to be near, and we always want you to care.

I am a subsequent child, and I have a subsequent child. I know.

~~~~~~~~~

Some things for others to know:

- I want you to remember my baby, the baby who died. I want you to recognize that the hardship of grief I am enduring is because I've been blessed with the role of mother and that I did, in fact, give birth to a baby. My baby.

- When you mention my baby, it is healing. If I cry, if I smile, if I seem cool – however I respond – it is healing.

- I am heartbroken because I am missing out on so many lovely things with my baby. When you call my baby by name, when you speak to me about my child, you are giving me something back.

- My experience is different than anyone else's. My journey is different than anyone else's. It is my journey. I'd like you to walk it with me and we can share what we see together – I do want you to point out what you see in me and around me. I don't want you to blindfold me and tell me where I need to step.

- The death of my baby is not exactly the same as the death of anyone else. We can share in our common denominator only if we don't use that as a means of forging or expecting each other to mourn a certain way.

- Joyous occasions, like the birth of another child, still are subsequent to the death of my child. There are no replacements – of my deceased child, or of the feelings I have for him.

- I am thankful for the life of my child, however brief, and for the reality of my child, which is eternal. I am humbly grateful for the things I have learned through his death and because of his death. Help me honor the reality of my child by remembering the day he was born, and the day he died.

- A pregnancy loss is still a birth, and is still a birthday. It is recurrent. It is annual. I want you to remember the day with me. As I recall the tiny person I saw, I will feel love for that child. This feeling is right and is intended to be shared. I will also feel sadness for the love I haven't been able to lavish onto that child. This feeling is also right and is intended to be shared. I'd like to share it with you, but more than that, I'd like you to share it with me. I'd like for you to initiate conversation – I'd like you to tell me that my baby's short life was important to you, and that my baby's eternal reality is important to you.

- Please remember my baby's important dates, just as you remember my other children's dates. Here is a nice card you can give me as I honor my baby's stillbirthday through the years.

- I'd like you to remember that I am still adjusting to my new life – my subsequent life – and I'd like you to offer me grace and forgiveness as I stumble on this journey.

- I have offered you grace and forgiveness as you've stumbled in the things you have done and said, and failed to do and say, to me. It is sometimes excruciating to do so, because I am adjusting to this new life and need caring for, but I do. If you are not sure of how to care for me, ask. I have answers to your questions.

- I am not alone in the way I feel about this subsequent life. One mother sends a plea to her loved ones to just say something to validate the reality of her child, while another challenges those who seek to shape the path of bereaved parents. And thousands more find their way here, to stillbirthday, because they, too, want to learn how to make sense of this new, subsequent life.

Irish Twins

When two babies are born nearly a year apart, they are said to be Irish twins. This happens when one baby is conceived three months after the other was born.

I already have one set of Irish twins. The older of the two is going to be three years old, and the younger is heading to be a two year old.

At first, they were 5 clothes sizes apart; while one was wearing 0-3 months, the other wore 9-12 month clothes. One was very much a brand new baby, while the other was a toddler. Today, I can manage to get them both to wear the same sized clothes, although one is exactly a head taller than the other. They get jealous and fight with each other. When one cries, the other cries louder. When one laughs, the other comes running to see what all the fun is about. They push each other down, wrestle each other, and they hug and snuggle each other too. They love each other.

My newest baby is also an Irish twin. She was born in April, and is the brand new baby in our home. Yet, she is a totally different kind of Irish twin. She and her Irish twin will never be mistaken for fraternal twins when I go grocery shopping or when I take the children to the park. She will not have the same competition to cry louder than the sibling immediately older than her. The two of them will not squeeze into our little children's couch, one pulling a blanket over the other ones lap, to snuggle with their sippy cups together and watch a cartoon.

You see, last April, I gave birth to my miscarried baby.

There is a person missing from our family in our family photos. There is a carseat missing in our car. There is a missing stack of folded laundry, there is no leaky sippy cup dribbling on the floor where one should be, there are no memories of scooting, rolling over, lifting his head, tasting his first solid food, wrapping his tight little hand around his grandma's finger or smiling big for his daddy.

There is an ache in my heart where fondness should be. And yet there is hope also, where presumption would surely have otherwise resided.

My heart, and my life, are forever filled with an ache and a hope that would have never otherwise been.

I should have been pregnant with my miscarried baby until November 2011.

I became pregnant with my daughter in July 2011.

What is it like to share a pregnancy – to share time that belonged to another of my babies?

It was lonely – shortly after my natural miscarriage, I took a home pregnancy test to confirm that it was in fact, negative. It is a terrible feeling to long for him, to miss him, to dread seeing the one, lonely line on that test, and yet knowing that the single line meant that my body had safely completed the birth of my tiny baby; to see so simply and matter 0f factly that to the rest of the world it was all over, and to know that in my heart, life without the presence of this child had only just begun.

It was angering -having to face a perfectly timed menstrual cycle, exactly 28 days following the miscarriage. To see that my body could naturally, instinctively, do what it was supposed to do, and yet it couldn't protect my sweet child – I felt like my body had cheated me.

It was confusing – when I saw the two pink lines for the first time with this pregnancy, where they should have remained with the former one, was bittersweet. I was not expecting to be nor was I trying to get pregnant. My heart was constantly challenged from the months of July to November, as I wondered what it would be like – how could I possibly prepare myself emotionally – if I not only experienced a second loss, but during the same time that I would have still been pregnant with my first miscarried baby?

It was humbling - these two babies could not have both lived here on earth. While traditional Irish twins are born a year apart, it is because the second is conceived three months after the birth of the first. It would have been virtually impossible for me to give birth to one child in November 2011, and the other in April 2012. God knows when we will be born - each of us. He knew when my miscarried baby would be born. He knew also when my daughter would be born. Neither of these births are an accident or outside of His purposes. They are both important. So while I know of the impossibility of both of these children living here on earth, I am confident in the hope that one day they both will in fact reside in eternity together. As impossible as it is for me to have my 5 children here, it is most certain that all 5 are made in the image of God Himself, have purposes, and have the opportunity to enter Heaven. In fact, one is already safely there.

It was a gift – God picked the timing. In the same month that my miscarried baby would have been born, November 2011, I also learned the gender of this baby, my first daughter. It was a gentle, pleasing buffer from the heartbreak, the agony, the despair that overcame my heart.

It was a challenge – as if I hadn't grown enough through the experience of losing my child, of first laboring and delivering and then burying my dead baby, I mentally prepared for facing April 2012. April, the month that held the first anniversary – the first "angelversary" – the first stillbirthday of my miscarried baby. April, the month I discovered that my baby was dead. The month I saw him, motionless on the ultrasound monitor. The month I prayed desperately, deeply, for the most important miracle of my entire life – "Please God, please, give a flicker of life. Please let him stir. Please don't tell me he is gone." The month I understood that God didn't ignore me, even though His reply seemed to be only silence – eery, overwhelming, my-life-will-never-be-the-same-again silence. The month that I was told that my dead baby didn't have value and that I could discard of him as I wished. The month I waited for labor to begin, the month I hated myself, the month I dreaded what the end of labor would bring. The month I knew I would face my dead child. The month I met him – saw his perfectly formed, tiny body. Counted his miraculously beautiful toes. Cried over him. Folded him into his final, miniscule bed, drove to the cemetary, saw the hole in the ground. The hole that would hold my child.

Yes, this very same month, only one year later, is when I planned and prepared for the birth of my miscarried baby's younger sister. I planned to experience labor again, anticipated what the labor would bring, hoped for who I would meet at the end of it. It is the month that I anticipated counting toes again and marvelling at God's perfect design. It is the month I hoped for what the end of labor would bring. The month I knew I would face my dear child.

Would God give me this child, to enjoy in this lifetime? Would I be able to hear her crying, bring her to my breast for comfort? Would I clean her tiny little poopies and snuggle her in warm pajamas? Would we need the carseat? Would a grave hold her, or would her mother?

It is the month I knew I would need to be submissive to God's will, and be ready for whatever outcome He ordained for our family. I would need to let God remain in control. I hoped – oh, how I hoped. I hoped and wished and prayed that this April would bring joy rather than more heartbreak.

I planned as though God would give our daughter to us in this life. And yet I accepted that His plans may be very different than that.

I didn't have the control. Much like the births of each of my other children, in fact including her Irish twin, I could only participate in the ways that have been permitted for me.

I prayed. I planned. I hoped. I submitted. I labored. And then, I met her…

Misconceptions of Miscarriage

I asked some of my fellow stillbirthday mothers to help me out with some misconceptions of miscarriage. This is our list, of misconceptions the people around us had – and said to us – in our darkest days of grief.

I'd like to build a misconceptions list of all pregnancy and infant loss experiences, so if you'd like, you can leave a comment with yours. Alternately, you can visit our article on bullying the bereaved, and use the special email address there.

In our heartbreak, we felt:

- Like a murderer.
- Like a bad mother.
- Like I couldn't even protect my baby…from myself.
- Like a failure.
- Like my husband must blame me.
- Like my husband should blame me.
- Like my husband wouldn't want to make love to me again.
- Shame at my body's desire to want intimacy again – feeling foolish for desiring sexual intimacy from my husband.
- Wondering if my husband is thinking about the loss during intimacy with me.
- Foolish to want to conceive again.
- Foolish to think I can conceive again.
- Foolish that my "womanhood" is so "incorrect" or "malfunctioned".
- Deep despair at the loss of effort it took to conceive – wasted time, money, effort.
- Self loathing – vengeance for my child's death, even if directed at self.
- Tempted to search for blame onto others, including my spouse, others, or God.
- Frustrated that even the platitudes were directed at my baby ("in a better place") or rushing me into some future projection of happiness ("you can try again") instead of focusing on my needs and the magnitude of the moment.
- Unable to perceive anything other than the current darkness, and so these platitudes about the future seemed like a foreign language.
- Pressure to move on, as if my body wasn't actually in a postpartum transition.
- Rejected.
- Weird.

In our heartbreak, we heard:

- It's over.
- You can forget.
- You should forget.
- You didn't love your baby, that's why you lost 'it'.
- Your life is easier with one less child to care for.
- It was God's will.
- You should consider yourself lucky.
- Your loss is easier than someone else's loss (loss of spouse, etc.)
- 'It' wasn't a real child.
- You shouldn't hurt mentally.
- You shouldn't hurt emotionally.
- You shouldn't hurt spiritually.
- You 'only' lost the idea of a baby.
- It's not real labor and childbirth.
- It's just a period.
- 'It's' just debris.
- 'It's' just products of conception.
- You are not a mother.
- God didn't approve of this baby.
- You didn't deserve to be pregnant.
- You should be thankful that you have your living children.
- You can just get pregnant again.
- You are lucky God changed His mind.
- You are lucky to not have a special needs child, that you were spared from this.
- This was God's will.
- It's your fault (your weight, your job, your stress, etc.)
- Adoption is an easy approach to parenthood.
- Silence.

Stillbirthday mothers, this is a very hurtful list. Just reading this hurts my heart. If in reading this list, you get stuck in pain, please, I ask you this. Please, get out a piece of paper and a pencil. Please go through every single one of these comments above, and read it in the OPPOSITE. Then, write down these OPPOSITE responses. It would look like this:

- I don't have to forget.
- God did not change His mind.
- I love my baby.
- Every loss is difficult – mine, and anyone else's.

Giving birth to our miscarried baby(ies) has taught us many things. It has stretched us to learn more about ourselves, about our feelings, about our values, about our patience, our forgiveness of others, and about our love.

I asked some stillbirthday mothers to expand on this with me. This is our list.

- It is good for me to honor my feelings.
- It is good for me to validate each of my children and speak about them as I choose to.
- It is good for me to include all of my children in conversations, in celebrations and in my family as I choose to.
- My experience is worthy of me defining how I choose to.
- I have the right to consider myself the mother to a miscarried child, for the rest of my life, and determine for myself how this role is an important one.
- My heart can hold love for people I have never seen.
- I am here, and I have a place, even when I feel lost.
- It is good for me to cry.
- It is good for me to laugh.
- Happy can remind me of sad. Sad can remind me of happy.
- I treasure today because tomorrow is unknown.
- I treasure my living children and other living loved ones, not because I was told to, but because I choose to.
- I want to grow and to improve areas of myself in honor of my child(ren).
- We all grieve differently.
- I am not grieving wrong.

Proclamation 5890 — Pregnancy and Infant Loss Awareness Month, 1988

October 25, 1988

By the President of the United States of America

A Proclamation

Each year, approximately a million pregnancies in the United States end in miscarriage, stillbirth, or the death of the newborn child. National observance of Pregnancy and Infant Loss Awareness Month, 1988, offers us the opportunity to increase our understanding of the great tragedy involved in the deaths of unborn and newborn babies. It also enables us to consider how, as individuals and communities, we can meet the needs of bereaved parents and family members and work to prevent causes of these problems.

Health care professionals recognize that trends of recent years, such as smaller family size and the postponement of childbearing, adds another dimension of poignance to the grief of parents who have lost infants. More than 700 local, national, and international support groups are supplying programs and strategies designed to help parents cope with their loss. Parents who have suffered their own losses, health care professionals, and specially trained hospital staff members are helping newly bereaved parents deal constructively with loss.

Compassionate Americans are also assisting women who suffer bereavement, guilt, and emotional and physical trauma that accompany post-abortion syndrome. We can and must do a much better job of encouraging adoption as an alternative to abortion; of helping the single parents who wish to raise their babies; and of offering friendship and temporal support to the courageous women and girls who give their children the gifts of life and loving adoptive parents. We can be truly grateful for the devotion and concern provided by all of these citizens, and we should offer them our cooperation and support as well.

The Congress, by Senate Joint Resolution 314, has designated the month of October 1988 as "Pregnancy and Infant Loss Awareness Month" and authorized and requested the President to issue a proclamation in observance of this month.

Now, Therefore, I, Ronald Reagan, President of the United States of America, do hereby proclaim the month of October 1988 as Pregnancy and Infant Loss Awareness Month. I call upon the people of the United States to observe this month with appropriate programs, ceremonies, and activities.

In Witness Whereof, I have hereunto set my hand this twenty-fifth day of October, in the year of our Lord nineteen hundred and eighty-eight, and of the Independence of the United States of America the two hundred and thirteenth.

Ronald Reagan

[Filed with the Office of the Federal Register, 11:13 a.m., October 26, 1988]

Unsubscribe Baby Mail

After a pregnancy loss or infant death, it can be very frustrating to continue to receive promotional coupons and information for baby related items through your mail, or to receive baby or pregnancy related emails in your inbox, or to have milestone updates that you won't reach with this pregnancy posted onto your social media.

How do you undo these things?

Direct Marketing Association is a mail preference service that helps you get the mail you want, and stop getting the mail you don't. Here is their contact information:
- Direct Marketing Association, Inc. 1615 L Street Washington, DC 20036
- 212-768-7277, ext. 1888

I have called them several times, and have sent them several emails using their contact form. I finally reached them, by asking for an operator.

Then, I registered, so that I could view the full listing of associated businesses. They are in four categories:
- catalogs
- magazine offers
- other mail offers
- credit offers (separate website)

I found nothing helpful under "other mail" which was where I went first. Then I went through the catalog and magazine listings. I found "American Baby", "Birthday Keepsakes", "Children's Wear Digest", "Early Childhood Manufacturer's Direct", and "Family Circle". These are the only companies listed with Direct Marketing Association (DMA). Other businesses, formula manufacturers, diaper companies, and cord blood banking companies are not currently listed.

If you would like to unsubscribe from any of those that are listed, you can register your account with DMA here.

When you register at websites or when you list for freebies, you are considered to be a customer, and they will send you any coupons or promotions they want. That means, going back to each website and unregistering (some moms wondered if somehow midwives or doctors sell personal information to product manufacturers. Through HIPAA, they can't do this).

So, ultimately, this leaves loss moms with three options:
1. Continue to get the mail for the baby we are no longer pregnant with. Some moms have the dads check the mail. Some moms rip and tear apart the coupons and ads as a time to release anger and frustration at not being pregnant anymore. Alternatively, some moms save some of the advertisements as something else that belongs to the baby.
2. Contact DMA, but this is largely ineffective.
3. Keep documentation of each baby registration, so that they can go back to each website to unsubscribe. For subsequent pregnancies, some mothers only register for sites with the quickest and simplest unsubscribing processes.
4. If you are in Europe, your Baby Mailing Preference Service can be helpful.

Poor Prenatal Preparation

What is a pregnancy loss?

"Miscarriages are labor, miscarriages are birth. To consider them less dishonors the woman whose womb has held life, however briefly."

~Kathryn Miller Ridiman, Midwifery Today 1997

The actual loss that a family experiences when it is called a pregnancy loss, even in the event of a very early miscarriage, may be considered to them to be the life of the anticipated and likely hoped for child.

When you consider that many mothers experiencing even a very early miscarriage consider it to be the death of a child (regardless of kind of miscarriage, and regardless of political views or religious beliefs), it certainly seems much more staggering, sobering, and even dare shall I say important than saying

"I had a miscarriage."

After a woman takes a pregnancy test and discovers that she is pregnant – nay, even before this, if she is intentionally trying to conceive – she surrenders herself to the role of mother.

She changes the way she eats, the way she views her world, the way she views herself.

She plans and prepares for her child.

A child, who will reflect her in many ways. A child who will carry on her husband's last name. A child who will bring joy to the family – who will continue the family.

This, and more, is not just lost, but taken, when she has a miscarriage. It is not by her choice. And nobody prepares her for it.

After she hears the news that her baby is dead or is going to die, she is thrust into an isolating world where no resources are available. Her pregnancy books, classes and Facebook pregnancy pages don't have information for her. Her doctor is limited in the things he can say.

Nobody talked about it, because nobody wanted to scare her -

- but, in the end, nobody prepared her, either.

Instead of information, resources and support, she is given platitudes, speculation, and abandonment.

She enters into a state of grief, likely compounded by postpartum depression, and nobody around her knows how to support her.

To change this, I asked a couple of pregnancy and birth professionals and advocates who have shared about pregnancy loss with their communities of readers to help me in finding ways for more professionals and advocates to open the door to discussing this extremely important topic.

As a pregnancy/birth professional/advocate, I encourage you to take the time to read what these amazing professionals have to say to you about how to approach the subject of loss and why it is so important that you do.

Please, also visit our Tips to Talking About It, so that you can learn how to open up this extremely important dialogue with your readers – the mothers who need this information.

I sought out hundreds of professionals and advocates, but only a small handful had replied back that they had ever discussed loss before. I asked them the following questions:

- What role do you have in pregnancy/birth information (a little intro)?
- How did you first broach the subject of pregnancy loss with your readers/community?
- What made you feel it was important?
- Was there anything that prevented you from sharing about it sooner? What was it?
- Did these fears or concerns present themselves after you did share about the subject?
- What unexpected problems did you find after you had broached the subject?
- Did it prove to be beneficial overall to discuss pregnancy/infant loss with your readers/community?
- Since sharing, have you discovered that there are topics/angles within the subject of pregnancy/infant loss that you feel unable to discuss (perhaps too graphic, related to birth choices involved in the loss, feel too uninformed about, too personal for yourself or possibly readers)?

Donna replied:

"I mainly run the Volusia County Birth Network and teach women and men about how a womans body works. To open up the subject of loss, I just put it in my bio on my website and put miscarriage info and links on my website. I shared a lot on my Facebook page and online forums. I felt it was important to share, becuase I had suffered loss and knew of other women who suffered loss and it seemed to be a subject people didn't talk about – **and I wanted to get it out in the open**. Lack of knowing how and where to share prevented me from discussing the topic sooner, but once I shared, I didn't find any unexpected problems and there have been no angles or topics within pregnancy loss that I have felt unable to discuss. It proved beneficial to share, because then I didn't feel so alone in my loss and grief."

Pamela Black added:

"I am a labor and birth doula, and a private birth educator (aspiring to do groups) in Denver. I began broaching the subject of loss by posting links to my Facebook page (which has a very small audience) and I've engaged in conversation with a "few" clients. I find the subject is a tough one. Most are very uncomfortable talking about death when they are focused on birth. One dad recently slammed his hand on the table when I brought it up and said "we need to move on." I discovered during their very long +30 hour labor at a hospital that ended in a Cesarean birth that he had a grandmother die due to anesthesia for surgery. He was totally freaked. **My biggest reason for discussing pregnancy loss is a desire for others to know there are resources and options available if they have the need.** I have found that couching it with "This most likely will not apply to you but you may find yourself one day able to take this information and be able to help a family member, a neighbor or a friend with these resources and encouragement." That usually helps them relax. I also talk about nilmdts in addition to stillbirthday. A little personal history: My first exposure to death was my 53 year old grandmother very unexpectedly died and I was devastated – due to family circumstances she was the one person I had bonded with the most as an infant. Then I had a miscarriage in 1974 and in 1976 had a 17 year old brother killed in a motorcycle accident. His death devastated my mother's life and therefore has impacted the rest of the family. Since then I have had many relatives, friends, co-workers, etc. die. As far as my own experience with miscarriage I openly grieved the loss in 2005 when through an "honoring life" ceremony I named him, acknowledged the profound impact his life had had on me over the years and received a "Life Certificate" that to this day means a lot to me. All that to say, I feel familiar with death and its seeming finality now escapes me. Where there was once devastation and confusion I can only find in me peace and assurance that everything is just as it's supposed to be. I've learned that reality is kinder than my imagination and I know God to be completely in control and deeply caring. I can only find in me acceptance and a surrender to a bigger picture that I believe will someday be revealed and perfectly understandable. Till then I don't need to know why, I trust. I have been a doula for 4 years and at a birth with fetal demise once. I sat, I listened, I cried, I hugged, I held her baby, I encouraged, I prayed … That is all I can do and because of God's amazing grace I feel honored to have played that small role in her life and in the life of the little one. I don't presume it was bigger than or more meaningful than what friends and family or even hospital staff may have done. I do think that I am doing my part and that is quite enough. I was also honored to be a birth with a couple who had had one miscarriage and one stillborn prior to. There was a silence when the baby was born and she didn't cry right away while the doctor was taking a little longer than mom was comfortable with and mom anxiously asked "Is she alive?" and at just that moment she cried and both parents exclaimed (and I cry at the memory) "She's alive, she's alive!" They now have three children.

Dr. Pauline Dillard continued:

"I am the executive director of the Dunamas Center where we do premarital and marriage counseling as well as childbirth education that is Christ centered, heart connecting and marriage focused. I was a birth educator and childbirth assistant for 12 years before going to graduate school in psychology. Currently my counseling work includes working with those who have had traumatic birth experiences and pregnancy loss. The main place we discuss pregnancy loss is our Choices for a Discerning Childbirth, when we discuss life issues that affect how people approach birth. However, I am currently getting more referrals from birth professionals and other counselors with regard to pregnancy loss and trauma, and will be doing more writing on the topic in the future. **Pregnancy and birth in all forms and outcomes impacts who we are as women, wives and moms.** It is a fundamental core part of who we are. I have also, always comfortable being with those in loss and trauma. I began with a particular interest in how pregnancy loss impacts the way couples would approach subsequent pregnancies and birth plans, and I wanted to help them to be confident and open to what God might have for them, and not be caught up in fear and pain when it came to future pregnancies and birth. I never faced any problems to discussing pregnancy loss. Many women are relieved to have someone to talk to who accepts their depth of loss and grief, and helps them walk through their pain and regain their footing. In fact, most of my counseling clients are relieved that I have background in natural birth and can ask them about the birth process (if it was a stillbirth), and affirm their choices, and can discuss pregnancy A & P as it might be related to a pregnancy loss. I am also able to help them with what questions they might want to explore with a care provider in the future, or if they still have questions about what happened that they may not have thought of. I am also quite open about anything they may want to talk about and can ask them hard questions without making them feel judged or put down. I don't have any current material on our web site specifically about pregnancy loss, but we will be adding a list of books and web sites that might be helpful. I will also be adding the topic to things I cover in counseling, and how we work with those who have had a pregnancy loss, or infertility issues, when it comes to subsequent pregnancies."

Ilise noted:

"I run a small blog and a couple of pages and a group on Facebook that are about pregnancy and birth. I can't remember when I posted for the first time about pregnancy loss, but it would have been within the last six months. Many women suffer from the loss of babies during pregnancy and birth and I've known friends and family that have, too. **I always feel so helpless when wanting to help them, but I know they feel pain that they don't always share and they don't always have many places to turn for understanding**. I don't think anything really made me question sharing. Even though I know some pregnant women are hesitant to read about loss while expecting, I still felt it was important to share to give them and others the chance to decide that for themselves. I don't really think anyone has vocally been upset by my sharing on loss. Someone once said that they wouldn't read it right then because they were expecting, but they would keep it in mind for later. Those who have commented, have said that it is helpful and healing to have a place of understanding and information."

Jen (vbacfacts.com) replied:

"I am a mom who manages a website on birth options after a cesarean where I share interesting or hard to find information. When I experienced a miscarriage at 7 weeks I wrote about it. 18 months later, I decided to share it via the website. Sometimes people can find comfort knowing that someone else understands their pain. Knowing friends who had also miscarried was helpful to me. I decided to share my story publicly so that other women might "know" someone who had experienced it. And for those that had not experienced miscarriage, for them to understand that women might still be in mourning months later even as they mother their children. The pain just doesn't go away when the bleeding stops. It proved to be beneficial to share. People don't often leave comments at my site, but the comments left when I shared about loss were very touching. I will include just a few that were shared:"

"Thanks for sharing. I've had 3 m/c and have 2 live children. It doesn't get easier, each loss is unique and painful. You're so right about how others act as if if never happened…**maybe stories like this will start to change that**."

"I have also chronicled my miscarriage experiences at my blog. And I talk very openly about my miscarriages and what my current pregnancy means to me. I try and present it in a way that people won't really feel sorry for me. I'm pretty open about it with the college students. They need to know that it is likely that they or someone they care about will experience miscarriage."

"Funny reading this from you this week. I miscarried about a month ago, a close friend miscarried about 2 weeks ago and another dear friend lost her little one this week. Its been quite an emotional rollarcoaster…trying to move through fresh grief and having the scab ripped open over and over again while trying to be a shoulder to cry on for others. Why is it so hard to talk about in our society? Why is it something we don't talk about, we're supposed to just forget it, accept it was fate and that's all. Thank you for reminding me that I- and many other women- aren't alone."

Please, also visit our Tips to Talking About It article that serves to work in conjunction with this one, so that you can learn how to open up this extremely important dialogue with your readers – the mothers who need this information.

In Twenty Minutes

In twenty minutes, a mother who has been laboring, in pain, terror, disbelief and anguish, will give one final push, and her silent, stillborn baby will be born.

In twenty minutes, a father, shocked, in horror and in terrible amazement, will watch as his lifeless child, perfect but still, is carefully swaddled.

He will watch as the doctor awkwardly and uncomfortably asks his distraught, grief stricken wife if she wants to hold this unmoving bundle of bleach smelled blanket and lifeless form.

The mother, wet from tears, sweat and blood, will be shaking, broken, overwhelmed, and will, with uncertainty, receive her baby in her arms. Both parents will feel ill-prepared and terribly alone.

In twenty minutes, this baby's older brother, a surviving sibling, will face weeks, maybe months of distraction and mood swings from his parents. He will wonder why mom is crying, or shouting, or throwing things for no reason. He will wonder why dad doesn't come home from work on time anymore or why he yells at him or his mom or why his dad retreats so often to tinker in the garage.

Yes, in fifteen minutes now, an ill-prepared loved one will soon tell this mother not to worry, because at least she has the older child.

Still another ill-prepared loved one will think to tell the parents that they can try again.

The distraught father will try to protect the mother from the mounting pain, anger, confusion and devastation. He will try to minimize his grief in an effort to minimize hers.

The baby who is born will not need a carseat. Returning home from the hospital, the birth will be unmarked by visitors bringing the family a warm meal.

Verily, in twelve minutes, a volcano of emotion, tension, and destruction will be brewing in these parents hearts.

The mother will wonder why everyone she knows and loves are demanding her to be so unloyal to her feelings of sadness and loss.

She will turn against those she loves as she retreats internally, trying to lick her own wounds while filling with resentment at being ignored and overlooked.

The surviving sibling – remember him? In ten minutes, he will not know it, but the family plan to attend church this Sunday will be vanished.

After a weekend of hiding quietly in his bedroom, listening to the sounds of wailing, hushed whispers and shouting from his parents, he will return to school on Monday, confused and lonely. He will wonder if his friends think he is weird, if his parents were bad, or if he somehow hurt his mom and killed his little sister.

He will begin to wonder if his parents love him. Or if they even should.

It is true; in five minutes, each person in the family will question God, will question life, will question purpose.

They will feel that others around them are rushing them to move on and forget. Forget that their child is not alive.

They will feel that others around them don't want them to count their child. That because nobody else knew their child, that their child doesn't count.

These parents, this mother and father, will look upon that bundle wrapped in a hospital blanket, and will wonder if they should push it away.

They will imagine – for just a moment – that pushing that bundle away, not looking, not touching, will help them move on faster.

Will help them forget. People they know will reflect this sentiment, time and time again, in the months and years to come.

But in three minutes, their hearts will be so heavy that they won't be able to move. They will be held there, in that moment, holding their lifeless baby.

In the United States alone,

- 600,000 mothers endure pregnancy loss through miscarriage
- 26,000 mothers endure pregnancy loss through stillbirth (source)

71 mothers today will give birth to a stillborn baby. 71 families will be changed forever, their spiritual health, relational health, marital health and even physical health will all be threatened. Illness and injury manifesting as silenced grief will affect each member of the family, causing time off of work, time out of school, and time stolen from family bonding. All 71 of these families need to know that they are not alone. That there is hope. That there is healing. That there is stillbirthday.

Every twenty minutes a stillborn baby is born, in the US alone.

It is happening,

right now.

Tell your loved ones, your co-workers, your neighbors, your medical providers, your religious leaders, that pregnancy loss is still birth.

That the birth experience is only the beginning of a lifelong process of living in grief, a lifelong quest to make sense of it and to find your place within it. That even the earliest miscarriage deserves to be honored as the birth, and the death, that it is. Tell them, tell them now:

A pregnancy loss is still a birthday.

www.stillbirthday.com

An Optional Activity

Drawing from the Well

We learned in chapter one a little about becoming a well. It is when we become a well, when we become deep and become still, that we can mirror back to the mother the validation she deserves and ultimately, provide the opportunity for the richest healing.

Learning how to become the well is not something that is academic. It is less about logic, thinking and knowledge (although these are involved) and more about transparency, about authenticity, about vulnerability and about a shared humanity.

Supplies:

For this activity, you'll need something to draw a nice circle, and have crayons ready.

This is an emotionally challenging activity, so it is helpful to have at least one support person on standby to help you unpack the feelings this activity might bring. Calling a very trusted friend or family member now, to let them know that you are engaging in what may be an emotionally challenging activity and that you might need their love afterward, is a great idea.

Getting Started:

We'll begin this activity – which is optional and not required – by reviewing some statistics:

- 1 out of every 6 American women has been the victim of an attempted or completed rape.
- 44% of rape victims are age 18 years and under.
- Victims of rape are 3 times more likely to suffer from depression, 6 times more likely to suffer from PTSD and 26 times more likely to abuse alcohol.
- Rape may or may not also cause pregnancy.
- 1 out of every 5 American girls has been the victim of child sexual abuse.
- "Non-contact sexual abuse" can include pornography, exposure and voyeurism.
- Children in broken homes (divorce or absentee parent) have a higher statistical chance of child abuse.
- Every 9 seconds a woman in the US is beaten.
- 10 million children witness domestic violence annually.
- Domestic violence is the leading cause of injury to women.
- Divorce rates vary by age, with the higher statistics being toward younger married couples – children of divorced families can be at higher risks of engaging in risky behaviors including sexual intercourse and drug or alcohol use.
- Every minute an American mother endures a miscarriage, and every 20 minutes an American mother endures a stillbirth (1 in 4 American mothers have endured pregnancy loss).

While the correlation of these statistics might not be clear to you yet, consider the following words:

- Betrayal
- Abandonment
- Abuse
- Humiliation
- Rejection
- Shame
- Fear
- Anger
- Depression
- Jealousy
- Emptiness
- Theft, Robbery, Stolen
- Yearning
- Neglect

Now, go back and read through that list of emotional words again, slowly, deliberately, each time thinking about yourself:

- As a child
- As a parent
- As a professional

Were you hurt as a child? Did you witness your mother or another woman being attacked? As a parent, have you faced divorce? Have you endured domestic violence?
As a professional, have you served a family and witnessed signs of domestic violence or abuse on women or children?

As a student doula studying birth & bereavement, are you afraid?

Have you been searching for healing?

As we each ache for emotional needs to be met, sometimes seemingly impossible gaps to be filled or restoration to be witnessed, we each, intrinsically, are worthy of receiving healing. Though we often find ourselves parched of refreshment, something deep within your own soul holds a hidden treasure of wisdom just for you to uncover. It may be spiritual in nature. It might be that a change in your nutritional habits can restore your physical health. Perhaps it's simply a whispered invocation to celebrate, rather than fear, being part of a community, and to trust, really trust, maybe for the very first time in your entire life, adult life or career, that you are in fact, not alone.

Getting Pregnant Again

This article serves to provide support resources for mothers and families who are currently pregnant after having endured a previous pregnancy or infant loss. Please also visit our Rainbow Birth Plan for information on planning the birth of your "subsequent/rainbow" baby.

It is extremely important to be aware that a subsequent pregnancy can likely bring with it heightened fears and anxieties. Having a Sacred Circle or blessingway can be a treasured way to celebrate this pregnancy.

If you are not yet pregnant with your subsequent pregnancy after loss, you might fill this time with love and rich healing. We have resources in our fertility challenges section on such subjects as conscious conception and pre-conception planning and bonding.

As you read this article, you can also listen in on a radio show with Heidi Faith (the founder of stillbirthday and author of The Invisible Pregnancy), Franchesca Cox (the founder of Still Standing magazine and author of Celebrating Pregnancy Again) with radio show host Gena Kirby (founder of Progressive Parenting):

Listen to internet radio with ProgressiveParenting on BlogTalkRadio

Please join us at our sister website, run by our doulas, at www.birthdiversity.net.

Many mothers consider subsequent pregnancy after loss to be a "rainbow" pregnancy, or they wait until this live baby is born and then refer to him or her as a "rainbow" baby. We talk about ways of incorporating special keepsakes and meanings into your Rainbow Birth Plan here at stillbirthday (see the end of this article for the link). Having a Boudoir Maternity photo session that includes rainbows, a memorial tattoo or other keepsake can be a way of facing challenges of discovering our inherent beauty and joy in a subsequent pregnancy.

Some things to consider in subsequent pregnancy:

- While there seems to be variability in professional opinion on the best time to try to conceive again following a pregnancy loss, many professionals recommend allowing one subsequent menstrual cycle to pass, to help ensure the uterus is clear of any fragments, possibly from the placenta.
- Parents need to be empowered to make pregnancy decisions on their own timeline. They already feel like they have lost so much power over what has happened to them.
- Mothers who conceive quickly may have a tendency to believe that the new baby will help to repair a lot of the expectations lost with the previous baby's death. Moms who are due around the time of their previous baby's anniversary (stillbirthday) are at particular risk of experiencing such feelings (1995 Child Bereavement Trust, UK).
- Other studies suggest that getting pregnant right away may allow the strongest of grief feelings to dissipate sooner.
- Guarded emotions, heightened anxiety, a tendency to mark off time by waiting for particular pregnancy milestones to come and go, and a need to seek out or avoid particular behaviors are common ways of coping with pregnancy after a loss (Syracuse University, 1999). This is true whether or not the mother has sought out, learned, and has attempted to or is working through medical reasons for her losses.
- Support groups can be very helpful in providing support to women going through pregnancy after a loss. They can help them to recognize that the others are going through the same experience, remember the babies who have died, learn new coping skills, and begin to relate to their living babies. Please see our article on various websites, including online groups.
- Bereaved parents who subsequently give birth to living children need to consider the place of the stillborn or miscarried child in the family and the relationship of the children who were born before the stillborn/miscarried child to those who arrive afterward.
- Loved ones may respond differently to the subsequent pregnancy than the mother. While the mother may be anxious and fearful, loved ones may pressure her to move on, forget her deceased child, and only celebrate her current pregnancy. Alternately, the mother may be feeling joyful at a subsequent pregnancy, only for loved ones to feel weary and blame the mother for getting pregnant again.
- Fear can present itself in many ways in subsequent pregnancy: fear of losing another child, fear of announcing the pregnancy, fear of betrayal toward the deceased child, fear of celebrating pregnancy, fear of the experiences of childbirth. Fear of the experiences of childbirth can include: remembering the last time her body gave birth, fear of contractions, fetal heart monitoring, crowning, and the moments immediately after birth.
- The challenges of balancing bereavement with joy often don't end with the birth of a live subsequent pregnancy, but just as in NICU grief, mothers of subsequent living children can face many experiences and seasons that remind them all over again of what all was lost at the death of their child: the same is true for fathers. Our Rainbow Birth Plan also includes information about our Rainbow Milk campaign.

Aspects of the above information are borrowed from the work of Ann Douglas, Author, Speaker of Canadian Foundation for the Study of Infant Deaths Converance from the Still Unanswered, Always Remembered slideshow (22)

Other helpful ideas:

- ■ Read other stories from stillbirthday, including subsequent pregnancies AND subsequent "rainbow" BIRTH stories!
- ■ You might also decide to include your baby who died in your subsequent pregnancy announcement. Here is one idea of how to do this. You might include the names of all of your family, a special keepsake, or a rainbow somehow.
- ■ Read our article "Your Subsequent Pregnancy" which has an invitation for you to share your experiences here at stillbirthday
- ■ Some mothers feel reservation about sharing the news of their subsequent pregnancy for fear that either she or others will be waiting for "bad news" to follow. Consider if it is more important to prevent having to retract the good news, or if it is more important to have support around you to reinforce the joy and encouragement of the pregnancy and to have "just in case" for emotional support if you do experience another loss. This is a personal decision that needs to be discussed with your husband.
- ■ Consider purchasing an iBirth app, Positive Pregnancy app, Sprout app or other similar device to give you updates on your pregnancy and other helpful features like an app-to-keepsake-book.
- ■ Consider using a fetal heart monitor at home.
- ■ Visit Count the Kicks
- ■ Consider using a fetal kick count chart.
- ■ Discuss your fears with your provider (midwife or OB).
- ■ Because of health concerns related to Dopplers and ultrasounds, consider asking your provider about MaterniT 21 testing as a possible alternative.
- ■ If you are considering purchasing or renting an at-home Doppler, there are organizations that can help you, such as Beats for Bristol. Please, consider discussing the use of one with your provider, including any possible risks of harm or health to your baby, by misusing or overusing the product.
- ■ our threatened miscarriage has some tips that may be helpful
- ■ facts/stats on pregnancy loss can be assuring
- ■ there are some natural fertility items such as stones, charms, and books in our keepsake list.
- ■ MotherPrayer is a spiritually diverse and supportive book.
- ■ Many mothers feel more comfortable in their subsequent pregnancies after they've reached two milestones: reaching the second trimester, and reaching the same gestational age at which they previously experienced a loss. Finding comfort and joy even during this "waiting" is important.
- ■ The hormones of pregnancy can serve to magnify hidden feelings. Pregnancy can also serve to magnify the feelings of grief. If you feel that you are experiencing heightened loneliness, anger, or dread, consult your provider along with your doula, and consider utilizing our long term support resources or joining our mentorship program.
- ■ Some mothers prefer to plan a more medicalized birth for susequent pregnancies, in an effort to prevent a loss. Please discuss these plans and your reasons for them with your provider.
- ■ Some mothers experience emotional dystocia during the labors of their subsequent children – an otherwise unexplainable delay during the birthing process, which may be contributed to fears or memories of delivering a miscarried or stillborn baby.
- ■ Consider using the Farewell Celebrations suggestions at any time after your loss and the Long Term Support resources to work through any residual fears and anxieties.

Get Connected

- ▪ Consider partnering with one of our mentors who can provide emotional encouragement through this time.
- ▪ Any of our highly trained SBD doulas would be honored to work with you through this pregnancy and birth as well. Our doulas know how to work with medically involved births, can lower the chances of unnecessary interventions, and can help you work through fears that may be prompting you to seek a more medicalized birth. SBD doulas can also help you incorporate very special, personal and meaningful ideas into your Rainbow Birth Plan.
- ▪ Hosting a Mothers Workshop can be a great way to address the complex feelings of pregnancy after loss.

Please join us at our sister website, run by our doulas, at www.stillbirthday.info.

Special books to help bring encouragement during this time

- ▪ The Invisible Pregnancy - a helpful book prior to getting pregnant again
- ▪ What am I Thinking? written by Karen Kleiman
- ▪ Celebrating Pregnancy Again written by Franchasca Cox.
- ▪ Finally, if it is needed, we have special information on having multiple losses

Rearing Living Children SBD Resources:

▪ Holding Umbrellas

Please join us at our sister website, run by our doulas, at www.stillbirthday.info. Stillbirthday provides resources and birth plans for every miscarriage and stillbirth experience.

Getting pregnant again after you've endured pregnancy & infant loss is often referred to as a "rainbow pregnancy". A "rainbow birth" might also be one in which a surviving multiple is born.

Here at stillbirthday, we know that there are five seasons a family deserves support through:

▪ Pregnancy/Prior to Birth
▪ Birth
▪ The Welcoming
▪ The Farewell
▪ Healing Journey

While on your healing journey, you may become pregnant again. And this "subsequent/rainbow" pregnancy does not forfeit your grief. In fact, it can bring additional joys – and, additional fears, worries and hurts.

Pregnant Again

If you are "pregnant again", here is some birth planning information for your "subsequent/rainbow" pregnancy and birth:

- Please read our information on emotional support during a "subsequent/rainbow" pregnancy.

- Consider having a special blessingway – Sacred Circle.

- You're invited to explore how stillbirthday Supports Birth Diversity. Please join us at our sister website, run by our doulas, at www.stillbirthday.info.

Subsequent or "Rainbow" Birth Plan

1. Including Plan Definitions, Expectations & Alternatives

- What do the options you are considering for this birth mean to you? How are they influenced by your motherhood journey thus far? What will it mean to you if your options change during the course of your labor? How might the sensations of labor, birth and the Welcoming be similar or different from your last encounter with these experiences? Consulting with experts, professionals and loved ones of a variety of perspectives might seem intimidating and frustrating, but can prove to give you some great insight into the possibilities and the reasons for your choices.
- Creating a pre-planning journal can be a tremendous tool. This journal might include Love Letters to your baby who is not alive, it might include Love Letters to your baby you are pregnant with, and it might include thoughts you have along the way. Returning to your writing at a later time can help refreshen your perspective.
- There are many non-medical options that can be personal and wonderful for you – options that may either replace or work in conjunction to medical support, including your SBD doula. If you are planning a home rainbow birth, stillbirthday mothers invite you to read about their experiences, which include extremely important things to consider, challenges you may face, and healing you may encounter. A beautiful book entitled Dancing with the Midwives is worth it to check out. The author talks about her hospital stillbirth and her home subsequent birth.
- Again, our information on emotional support during a "subsequent/rainbow" pregnancy can prove tremendously helpful.
- This mother and newly adopted baby below, are bonding in a "recreated" waterbirth experience (click here for their story). It is never too late to facilitate bonding, even when birth plans include the most amount of medical intervention. Your love and your creativity can create an experience of love that is deeply meaningful and personal.

2. Including Support

- Consider hiring a Stillbirthday Birth & Bereavement Doula. This list includes SBD doulas and other birth professionals. SBD doulas do not only provide support for miscarriage and stillbirth, but SBD doulas are trained to provide support in all birth situations and experiences, including live births and including "subsequent/rainbow" births.
- Learning a bit about what we call "rainbow fatigue" can be helpful, which can carry some of the same traits as "baby blues".

3. Including Siblings

- You might include a symbol or a keepsake that represents your baby(ies) who died. You can visit our Claim the Space and our Still Together sections for keepsake/representing ideas.

4. Including Symbols

- You might include rainbows somehow into the birth setting: order a stillbirthday exclusive rainbow milk teether with special engraving! A rainbow colored receiving blanket, newborn hat, ink prints, leg warmers, onesie, wrap/carrier or other items.

5. Including stillbirthday

- You can share your birth story here at stillbirthday, as encouragement for other stillbirthday mothers. We have a section of writings entitled "Getting Pregnant Again"- which holds the reality of loss, life, hopes and fears in subsequent pregnancies, as well as our Rainbow Birth stories.

Sacred Circle

The Origin of Blessingways and Sacred Circles

While the name Blessingway is becoming more widely understood to mean a kind of "baby shower of spiritual gifts rather than physical ones", the origin traces to the Navajo tribespeople, and out of respect for their traditions, here at stillbirthday, we draw from the Blessingway term you might be familiar with, but then we point to our own name for our own interpretation of this beautiful event, coining the name Sacred Circles. This is quite appropriate as the burning zero candle is our trademarked image. Many of the events for our Sacred Circles are inspirations of Doran Richards of the Blessing God's Way website and resources.

I invite you also to visit our Loved Ones and Farewell Celebrations resources for even more suggestions in offering love to bereaved loved ones.

This is the first and only Blessingway specifically created to honor pregnancy, to honor the mother,

and to validate the very real life, and death, of your baby.

- The celebration will be a time of validating the mother and her mixed and real emotions, as well as a time to celebrate her very real child, even for the very short time the child is alive – in the womb or after birth.
- The celebration will be personal; there is no exact "one right way" to host one.

Tips to making this celebration successful for the mother:

- A Celebrating Pregnancy Blessingway, or, Sacred Circle is a time of intimate fellowship. The mom's closest friends and most special people should be all who are invited. Please keep the guest list less than about 16 people.
- The celebration might be in an inviting and soothing location, where the mom is comfortable being.
- It might include praying over the mother and her family as she faces the birth and death of her baby.
- It should include personalized gifts, brought by every person attending. These can include written scriptures, poems, or a letter, to be read aloud by the giver, to the mother, at the celebration. Other gifts may include: a journal, an inspirational book about infant loss, a handmade baby blanket, or a bead, specially chosen for the mother, and strung into a handmade necklace that the mother can wear – during the blessingway, and during birth in a subsequent pregnancy.
- Consider printing out special scriptures and quotes, on pretty paper, and use to fill the room with them. Consider also purchasing a Certificate of Life, or inviting the mother to do so. Collect these items at the end of the celebration, so that the mother can fill her home with these lovely, encouraging words.

- **It is important that each guest demonstrate the importance this baby has had on that individual. It is okay to cry. It is okay to say "I'm sorry". It is okay to give the mom a hug.**

- A tea candle might be lit after each gift is presented to the mother.
- Special, personal gestures of love toward the mother should be made during this celebration, including brushing her hair, putting flowers in her hair, and washing her feet with a lovely scent (lavender perhaps) and with warm, clean water. Touching the mother and singling her out in love is important. It should be decided prior to the celebration who will wash the mothers feet. This is a very personal, and very honoring, gesture.

- A special ceremony that includes wrapping the mother's womb, with gentle music playing, can be very honoring. The Womb Wrap we use in our Mothers Workshop is one very long piece of simple cloth. Each person in the circle takes turns wrapping the cloth around the mother, whispering a special mantra, encouragement or prayer to her. The wrap is not knoted. The cloth instead, rised and weaves and so each whispered prayer loops together, never ceasing, wrapping the mother in a continued message of love. In our Mothers Workshops, we also include a special warmth pad and we complete this portion of the ceremony with a brightly colored and breezy rebozo that jingles and sways gently as she moves. You can purchase this Womb Wrap to include in your Sacred Circle, and the mother can utilize it after every birth, during menstruation, and absolutely any time she needs to be wrapped in warmth and love.

- If this Sacred Circle is done during the mother's subsequent pregnancy, it might include a special red cord tied around each attendees (left) wrist. This cord is a reminder that there is a connection between the circle of attendees and to hold on through the pregnancy. During birth, this cord is cut from each person's wrists as a ceremonial ritual of release – release of fears, which can manifest during labor, and that it is time to open and birth.

According to the "Ask The Rabbi" column on the Ohr Somayach, Jerusalem website:

Wearing a thin scarlet or crimson string as a type of talisman is a folk custom among Jews as a way to ward off misfortune brought about by the "evil eye". The tradition is popularly thought to be associated with Judaism's Kabbalah.

The red string itself is usually made from thin scarlet wool thread. It is worn as a bracelet or band on the left wrist of the wearer (understood in some Kabbalistic theory as the receiving side of the spiritual body), knotted seven times, and then sanctified with Hebrew blessings.

A custom that is based on Torah ideas or mitzvoth may also have special segula properties on a smaller scale. Regarding the red string, the custom is to tie a long red thread around the burial site of Rachel, the wife of Jacob. Rachel selflessly agreed that her sister marry Jacob first to spare Leah shame and embarrassment. Later, Rachel willingly returned her soul to God on the lonely way to Beit Lechem, in order to pray there for the desperate Jews that would pass by on their way to exile and captivity. Often, one acquires the red string when giving charity.

Perhaps for these reasons the red thread is considered a protective segula. It recalls the great merit of our matriarch Rachel, reminding us to emulate her modest ways of consideration, compassion, and selflessness for the benefit of others, while simultaneously giving charity to the poor and needy. It follows that this internal reflection that inspires good deeds, more than the string itself, would protect one from evil and harm.

- Consider taking photographs of the celebration, to send to the mother, to remember her special celebration and fellowship.
- The celebration might close in a prayer over the ladies present and families represented, and over the meal that is to follow.
- The meal should consist of one item brought by each guest. Leftovers should be given to the mother to take home.

The focus of this celebration is to honor her as mom, to share feelings, and to encourage and uplift one another. The tone should be kept inspirational, validating and loving. You might invite a local SBD doula or Heidi Faith to help coordinate or guide your event.

Related: Mother's Workshop   Related: Mother Roasting

For more how to and photos: http://www.stillbirthday.com/2011/08/11/celebrating-pregnancy-blessingway/

General Stats & Info about Stillbirthday

Stillbirthday began on a free platform with free, printable birth plans for birth in every trimester and a free doula listing. Within the opening week talk was already escalating about a formal training to learn even more.

We reach 1 million visitors annually and the number is rising exponentially.

We have certified SBD doulas in several countries, including: US, Canada, Africa, Australia and Germany.

The website has been translated into multiple languages to serve families globally.

About the Training

We have scholarship and sponsorship programs, as well as network / partner / team building options.

Two demographics are seasoned birth professionals (doulas, nurses, midwives) and bereaved mothers with no academic training or professional experience.

Most of the seasoned birth professionals do not expect the training to impact them on a personal level. Most are surprised that it does, and to what level it does.

Most of the bereaved mothers are fearful that the worth of their child's legacy is conditional upon graduating the program.

The recidivism or immediate rollover repeat registration (into next subsequent training session) is between 30% – 40%, with a first time graduation rate as low as 10%-20%.

Most graduated SBD Doulas trailblaze to create programs in their communities, including speaking to local professionals and building local networks of strong SBD teams, as well as initiating the NICU ribbons program, Love Cupboards, seamstress teams, joining the SBD online continuing education opportunities (we never recertify) and more. This happens abroad as well.

From an SBD Survey

- 100% of all mothers interviewed in a stillbirthday poll published in 2012 indicated that obstetric/medical professional involvement directly influenced their interpretation of their experience and consequently, their journey beyond the immediate pregnancy and infant loss.

- 86% of those surveyed said that they wish they had had a trained SBD Doula in addition to their medical care team.

- 92% of those surveyed who indicated that they had a subsequent pregnancy indicated a combination of a heightened anxiety and anticipation of prenatal appointments.

Types of Loss

- By Gestational Age.

- By Meaning of Pregnancy Number (first boy, etc.)

- Chemical Pregnancy (miscarriage prior to ultrasound)

- Honoring Uncertainty

- Blighted Ovum

- Ectopic Pregnancy

- Molar Pregnancy

- Threatened Miscarriage

- Inevitable (or Incomplete) Miscarriage

- Missed Miscarriage (or "Silent Miscarriage")

- Complete Miscarriage

- Live Miscarriage

- Vanishing Twin/papyraceus

- Twins or More: one or more living

- Twins or More: none living

- Selective Reduction or Termination for Medical Reasons (TFMR)

- Recurrent Miscarriage (including fertility challenges/parenting options)

- Fertility Challenges

- Elective Abortion

- Stillbirth

- Difficult or fatal diagnosis in pregnancy

- NICU grief

- Living grief (grieving aspects of parenthood, related to children who are alive: includes birth trauma, adoption, surrogacy, menopause)

- Stewarding grief (emotional aspects of deciding to limit or inhibit fertility)

- Homebirth/ Out of Hospital Loss

- Neonatal Death
- Pregnancy Loss after Medically Assisted Conception (or grief after ART)
- Child Loss (toddlers to teens)
- Maternal Death
- Living Grief (NICU grief, surrogacy, fostering, adoption, birth trauma, stewarding grief)
- Bereaved Friends & Family including Siblings & Child Grief
- Bereaved Providers
- Getting Pregnant Again / "Rainbow Pregnancy"/ Rearing after Loss / Tandem Nursing Grief: Rainbow Milk
- Ending Fertility With a Loss

www.stillbirthday.com

More Unique Aspects to Consider

Based on our Library Collection

www.stillbirthday.com/library

- Adoption/ Foster/ Surrogacy Loss
- All Multiples All Newborns/ Diagnosis
- Blended Family
- Blighted Ovum/ Molar
- Child Death (infancy to adulthood)
- Dads
- Diversity (cultural, ethnic, faith, regional)
- Donating Decisions (organ, tissue, breastmilk)
- Ectopic Pregnancy
- Election Not Desire
- Ending Fertility With Loss & TTC Challenges
- Friends & Family (stories from loved ones perspective)
- Holidays (and the struggle to face them)
- Home Birth Loss/ Out-of-Hospital Loss
- Honoring Uncertainty (for mothers who believe they experienced loss but do not know for certain)
- Infertility/ Recurrent Loss (different from "ending with a loss", this section includes recurrent losses)
- Leap Day Losses (the calendar only honors this day once every 4 years. We honor this day every year.)
- LGBTQ+
- Live Miscarriage ("neonatal death" of babies born alive prior to "age of viability")
- Living Grief (includes adoption, menopause, or decision to end fertility, while still recognizing the pain of loss in this decision)
- Loss after ART (assisted reproductive technology)
- Loss after Rape or Abuse

- Military

- NICU Grief (the difficult journey of just the NICU)

- Poetry

- Prior to the 1990's (because every decade sees dramatic change in support)

- Provider Care (stories for and by providers: nurses, doulas, midwives)

- Siblings (stories & art for and by siblings, as well as general information that may support youth)

- Single, Separated or Widowed Parents

- Snowflake Babies (frozen embryos)

- Stewarding Grief (decision to end fertility but grieving)

- Teen Parents

www.stillbirthday.com

My Notes

About the Training

As we start a new class, inevitably friends and supporters of the SBD doula students want to have a peek, an inside view of what the student is learning, how the student is being challenged, and in what ways the student is being inspired. Here is a place for SBD students themselves, to comment and share a bit of their journey.

Week 1: fertility, pre-conception, conception, diversity in beliefs about pregnancy, birth and loss

Week 2: prenatal bonding, nutrition, partners, physiology of childbirth in every trimester

Week 3: medical support options during childbirth in every trimester

Week 4: non-medical support options during childbirth in every trimester, birth plans, building a doula bag & networking

Week 5: physical postpartum in all experiences, NICU

Week 6: emotional postpartum in all experiences, hormones, grief

Week 7: mourning, the emotional experience of the doula

Week 8: the practical, professional and business aspects of the doula

What is the SBD training?

"Stillbirthday's Birth & Bereavement Doula training is amazing. Heidi has created comprehensive materials that far exceeded my expectations and instilled in me a strong confidence to support loss parents during their darkest hour. The human touch she weaves into the training confirmed for me that I'd made the right decision in choosing stillbirthday for this experience."

-Jaime Hogan, part-time volunteer SBD

"Still Birth Day is an amazing program. I highly suggest ALL doulas take it, regardless of who else you trained/certified through."

-Shannon Sasseville, SBD trained doula

"Please know that I have learned so much more in this course than I had hoped and than I had learned in my five years of university. It has been an absolutely amazing honour to have been given the opportunity to meet so many wonderful women and to acquire all of this extensive knowledge. I cannot say enough about Stillbirthday and I am so incredibly thankful that my journey through grief led me to this opportunity. I truly feel that this is my calling and I will forever be indebted to you for all you do and for giving me the tools that I need to follow my dream. Thank you so much!"

-Jasmin Herchak, SBD student

"Stillbirthday is a refuge for the heart, a safe haven where unconditional love abounds, a place of solace. I am honored to be a SBD doula. My motherhood journey began with a pregnancy loss. The loss of my baby shaped me in very profound ways. It was out of this loss that I felt compelled to take the training and become certified to help other families in their time of grief and mourning. As a SBD doula I am able to support birth in any trimester with any outcome. At Stillbirthday a pregnancy loss is still a birthday. It is a community where resources can be found for birthing plans, farewell celebrations and bereavement support. When I had my miscarriage I did not know anyone who had suffered the same loss. My arms were empty, my eyes were full of tears and my heart was so very heavy. I sought comfort in my faith in God. I knew he was the creator of the life in my womb. 2 Corinthians 1:4 says He comforts us in all our troubles so that we can comfort others. When they are troubled, we will be able to give them the same comfort God has given us. It is my desire to comfort others in their time of need. Stillbirthday is like balm for the grieving soul. Stillbirthday has equipped me to walk out the desire of my heart in a tangible and meaningful way. If you are in need of compassion because you have experienced loss or if you are interested in becoming a birth and bereavement doula please visit www.stillbirthday.com a place where all are welcome and loved."

-Holly Lowmiller, SBD published at PaxBaby

"In my opinion, stillbirthday is one of the most rigorous available. Furthermore, the inclusion of miscarriage and stillbirth information provides a firm foundation for helping clients through unexpected outcomes."

-Summer Thorp-Lancaster, SBD student

"Many people don't understand the enormity of this training. It's 8 weeks (you have 12 to finish it) and it can be completely overwhelming. So many people NEED the 12 weeks to complete it. I have never taken training like this before. I would say it's close to an accelerated college course. Each week you have reading, assignments, and discussions. Some of the assignments involved making phone calls or visiting hospitals and/or funeral homes. In addition, there are 2 books reports and a community project.
You won't be disappointed. I know many people look down on online training but this isn't the same."

-Elizabeth Petrucelli, SBD and author of All That is Seen and Unseen

"I salute you Heidi for the brilliant work you have done to start Stillbirthday. It was a life changing course for me, and I hope I can now better serve the people that the Lord brings across my path. On behalf of all the other students and Doulas, thank you for everything you put into it. We can clearly see that all your heart is in this. Thanks for sharing so honestly and thanks for taking the lead in the field. Not only in the US, but also internationally. My life is so much richer with SBD in my life."

-Rechelle Vermaak SBD serving South Africa

What is an SBD Doula?

"Birth & Bereavement Doula: A birth doula is an essential part of a mother's support team during the childbearing year, especially during actual childbirth. A birth doula provides constant emotional and physical support, information, and promotes a loving, safe, non-judgemental environment for the mother and her family. Similarly, a bereavement doula goes further and provides families with constant support during one of the most difficult times of their lives. Bereavement doulas help families by facilitating healing through love, humility, and respect. It is important for families to feel unconditionally supported in the event of a loss, especially because there are often external factors that may make them feel as though they cannot express how they truly feel, thus hindering the healing process. Sometimes families do not have adequate family support or they feel as though their loved ones won't understand. It is important to serve these families in a way that helps them identify and address these feelings, and to be able to grieve in their own way to promote healing."

-Brandy Crigger, SBD student

"Doulas provide support and comfort that can make such a noticeable difference to birth mothers and the fathers too. Support during bereavement can be life changing. Memories of loss will be replayed over and over and will be remembered for a lifetime and will be grasped for something to hold on to. A doula's support can make the difference in those precious moments that will last a lifetime. At no other time in my life did I need support as much and at no other time was it as difficult to find. During loss the family is in shock it is hard to do basic life but at that moment you must make decisions you probably never considered before. To have the service of a doula to provide guidance, affirmation, preparation, and to justify feelings. To help remove fear so that the couple may bond with their precious child. This can make all the difference."

-Ashleigh Gipson, SBD student

My Notes

Websites & Resources

{born} photography - videographed our first international birth professionals workshop in Canada. The photos on the front and back cover are courtesy of the amazingly talented Calla Evans of {born} photography.

Give her page a like at - *www.facebook.com/bornbycallaevansphotography*

www.stillbirthday.com

www.stillbirthday.info

Doodles

www.stillbirthday.com

ABOUT THIS BOOK

This is simply a compilation of the most urgent and immediate support and resources that families may need in facing the earliest moments of birth and bereavement. As a resource for workshops and presentations, you may find that you can offer the information in this book to families you serve. You may also have found a word here just for your own heart.

Please do not copy or redistribute the content of this book.

This book is a compilation of selected pages of stillbirthday, based on those most frequently visited at the website. Because resources, research and information changes regularly, some of the details may become dated after publication. Please see your speaker for clarification and stillbirthday for the most updated content.

The core messages:
that every mother has a right to an informed decision to include a doula in her experience
that there are infinite spaces where birth and bereavement meet
that we have a collective responsibility to enter into those spaces with reverence and love, and
that a pregnancy loss is still a birthday

are legacies of love passed down to us through our children.

Please, visit stillbirthday for a much more comprehensive support – prior to, during and after birth in any trimester, and for support for the healing journey.

Presenter Name

Date

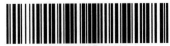

Made in the USA
Charleston, SC
25 February 2015